CONTENTS

INTRODUCTION

The Blue Zones Mediterranean Diet is known for its health and longevity benefits and the vibrant flavors found in regional staples like sun-ripened tomatoes, savory olive oil, fresh fish, and hearty whole-grain bread.

Whether you're new to this way of life or you grew up eating a Blue Zones Mediterranean Diet, The Blue Zones Mediterranean Diet Cookbook offers flavorful, heart-healthy dishes for everyone. Bring the Mediterranean Diet--from Italy and Greece to Morocco and Egypt, to Turkey and Lebanon--into your kitchen with more than 100 fresh, flavorful recipes. This comprehensive Blue Zones Mediterranean Diet Cookbook translates the famously healthy Blue Zones Mediterranean Diet for home cooks with a wide range of creative recipes; many are fast enough to be made on a weeknight, using ingredients available at your local supermarket.

The Blue Zones Mediterranean Diet isn't just a way of eating, it's a lifestyle—a complete approach to feeling your best both physically and mentally. The Blue Zones Mediterranean Diet Cookbook makes it easy for you to start and stay on the diet for long-term health.

Changing to a Blue Zones Mediterranean Diet is one of the most important decisions you can make to improve your health, boost energy levels, and also prevent chronic diseases.

People who follow the Blue Zones Mediterranean Diet have a longer life expectancy and lower rates of chronic diseases than do other adults.

And now you have a good chance to get The Blue Zones Mediterranean Diet Cookbook that can help you to save your time and cook super healthy meals.

Discover how this naturally healthy (and delicious) diet can help with heart health, weight management, and more. Dig into a variety of tasty options for everything from breakfast to dessert—all suited for two.

The Mediterranean Sea is surrounded by an extraordinarily diverse group of countries: Italy, France, and Spain to the north, Greece, Turkey, Israel, Lebanon, and Syria to the east, and to the south, the North African countries of Egypt, Tunisia, Morocco, Algeria, and Libya. This means that there isn't a single "diet" that encompasses the entire Mediterranean region—the spice-laden dishes of Morocco bear little resemblance to the lemon- and caper-laced cuisine of southern Italy. Rather, the Mediterranean diet is about what these cuisines have in common: a daily emphasis on vegetables and fruits, beans and lentils, whole grains, more seafood than meat and poultry, and heart-healthy olive oil. This is the essence of the Mediterranean way of eating and was our overriding principle when deciding what to include in this book.

Changing to a Mediterranean diet is one of the most important decisions you can make to improve your health, boost your energy levels, and also prevent chronic diseases. Science shows that eating more healthily helps you to live longer, it can also help the environment and to reduce the risk of getting sick.

The Mediterranean diet is a very simple style of eating and cooking. It doesn't involve a ton of rules, and it never sacrifices taste or nutrients. Features simple recipes, often rich in beans, vegetables, lean protein, whole grains, herbs, and spices.

My family and I have always loved to cook and experiment in the kitchen, and over the years we've moved more toward the Mediterranean diet. It's partly because of the research on its health benefits, which include lower rates of heart disease, diabetes, cancer, and depression. We also like our food to taste great too, and that's the main reason we've gone Mediterranean.

To help you start thinking about putting the Mediterranean diet into practice, we've compiled a list of recipes that we think work well together.

This book is also beneficial for those people who have wondered about the Mediterranean diet but had absolutely no idea where to start. This Mediterranean diet cookbook is looking forward to help people make changes in their life, starting with their diet.

If you want to start a Mediterranean diet but don't know exactly where to start, don't worry! This book is just for you. Here you can find everything so you can make this change easy and also enjoy it. Here you can find the answers to your questions, advice, and some techniques that you may need.

This cookbook gives you the opportunity to nourish yourself in a simple, affordable, and delicious way. Start cooking with these Mediterranean recipes today as making this change could save your life!

With this cookbook, you will enjoy simple and delicious Mediterranean diet meals that you will love and eat again!

Welcome to the Blue Zones Mediterranean Diet Cookbook lifestyle.

Enjoy!

BREAKFAST

Orange Cardamom Buckwheat Pancakes

PREP: 15 MINUTES • COOK TIME: 10 MINUTES • TOTAL: 25 MINUTES• SERVES: 2

Ingredients

½ cup buckwheat flour
½ teaspoon cardamom
½ teaspoon baking powder
¼ teaspoon baking soda
½ cup milk
¼ cup plain Greek yogurt
1 egg
½ teaspoon orange extract
1 tablespoon maple syrup (optional)

Directions

1.   Preparing the Ingredients

In a medium bowl, combine the buckwheat flour, cardamom, baking powder, and baking soda. In another bowl, combine the milk, yogurt, egg, orange extract, and maple syrup (if using) and whisk well to combine. Add the wet ingredients to the dry ingredients and stir until the batter is smooth.

2.   Cooking

Heat a nonstick skillet or a griddle over high heat. When the pan is hot, reduce the heat to medium. Pour the batter into the pan to make four 6-inch pancakes. Depending on the size of your pan, you may need to do this in four batches.

Garlicky Kale And Parsnips With Soft-Cooked Eggs And Pickled Onions (Instant Pot)

PREP: 22 MINUTEs • COOK TIME: 3 MINUTES • TOTAL: 45 MINUTES • SERVES: 4

Ingredients

12 ounces parsnips, peeled
2 tablespoons extra-virgin olive oil, plus extra for drizzling
4 garlic cloves, minced
2 pounds kale, stemmed and cut into 1-inch pieces
¾ cup chicken or vegetable broth
½ teaspoon table salt
4 large eggs
¼ cup Quick Pickled Onions
½ cup Lemon-Yogurt Sauce
1 teaspoon ground dried Aleppo pepper

Directions

1.   Preparing the Ingredients

Cut parsnips into 2-inch lengths. Leave thin pieces whole, halve medium pieces lengthwise, and quarter thick pieces lengthwise.

2.   Cooking

Using highest sauté function, cook oil and garlic in Instant Pot until fragrant, about 1 minute. Stir in half of kale and cook until slightly wilted, about 1 minute.

Add remaining kale and repeat. Stir in broth and salt, then add parsnips.

Lock lid in place and close pressure release valve. Select high pressure cook function and cook for 3 minutes.

Turn off Instant Pot and quick-release pressure. Carefully remove lid, allowing steam to escape away from you. Season kale and parsnips with salt and pepper to taste. Transfer to bowl and cover to keep warm. Discard cooking liquid in pot.

Arrange trivet included with Instant Pot in base of now-empty insert and add 1 cup water. Using highest sauté function, bring water to boil. Set eggs on trivet. Lock lid in place and close pressure release valve. Select high pressure cook function and set cook time for 3 minutes. Cook eggs for 2½ minutes (fully set whites with runny yolks) or 3 minutes (fully set whites with fudgy yolks). Turn off Instant Pot and quick-release pressure. Carefully remove lid, allowing steam to escape away from you. Using tongs, transfer eggs to separate bowl and place under cold running water for 30 seconds. Drain and peel eggs. Divide kale and parsnips among individual serving bowls. Top with pickled onions, yogurt sauce, and eggs. Sprinkle with Aleppo pepper and drizzle with extra oil. Serve.

Sunny-Side Up Baked Eggs With Swiss Chard, Feta, And Basil

PREP: 15 MINUTES • COOK TIME: 10 TO 15 MINUTES • TOTAL: 30 MINUTES • SERVES: 4

Ingredients

1 tablespoon extra-virgin olive oil, divided
½ red onion, diced
½ teaspoon kosher salt
¼ teaspoon nutmeg
⅛ teaspoon freshly ground black pepper
4 cups Swiss chard, chopped
¼ cup crumbled feta cheese
4 large eggs
¼ cup fresh basil, chopped or cut into ribbons

Directions

1.   Preparing the Ingredients

Preheat the oven to 375°F. Place 4 ramekins on a half sheet pan or in a baking dish and grease lightly with olive oil.

2.   Cooking

Heat the remaining olive oil in a large skillet or sauté pan over medium heat. Add the onion, salt, nutmeg, and pepper and sauté until translucent, about 3 minutes. Add the chard and cook, stirring, until wilted, about 2 minutes.

Split the mixture among the 4 ramekins. Add 1 tablespoon feta cheese to each ramekin. Crack 1 egg on top of the mixture in each ramekin. Bake for 10 to 12 minutes, or until the egg white is set.

Allow to cool for 1 to 2 minutes, then carefully transfer the eggs from the ramekins to a plate with a fork or spatula. Garnish with the basil.

Julene's Green Juice

PREP: 5 MINUTES • COOK TIME: NONE • TOTAL: 5 MINUTES• TOTAL: 5 MINUTES • SERVES: 1

Ingredients
3 cups dark leafy greens
1 cucumber
¼ cup fresh Italian parsley leaves
¼ pineapple, cut into wedges
½ green apple
½ orange
½ lemon

Directions
1.   **Preparing the Ingredients**
Pinch grated fresh ginger. Using a juicer, run the greens, cucumber, parsley, pineapple, apple, orange, lemon, and ginger through it, pour into a large cup, and serve.

Strawberry Basil Honey Ricotta Toast

PREP: 10 MINUTES • COOK TIME: 30 MINUTES • TOTAL: 40 MINUTES • SERVES: 2

Ingredients
4 slices of whole-grain bread
½ cup ricotta cheese (whole milk or low-fat)
1 tablespoon honey
Sea salt
1 cup fresh strawberries, sliced
4 large fresh basil leaves, sliced into thin shreds

Directions
1.   **Preparing the Ingredients.**
Toast the bread. In a small bowl, combine the ricotta, honey, and a pinch or two of sea salt. Taste and add additional honey or salt if desired. Spread the mixture evenly over each slice of bread (about 2 tablespoons per slice). Top each piece with sliced strawberries and a few pieces of shredded basil. Ricotta cheese is often overlooked unless you're making lasagna for a crowd. However, it's a great source of protein and full of calcium. It's also a nice, silky-smooth spreadable cheese that you can make sweet or savory for a meal or snack. Spread it on high-fiber whole-grain toast and top it with fruit. Perfect for a quick breakfast or afternoon snack.

Greek Yogurt Breakfast Parfaits With Roasted Grapes

PREP: 5 MINUTES • COOK TIME: 25 MINUTES • TOTAL: 30 MINUTES• SERVES: 4

Ingredients
1½ pounds seedless grapes (about 4 cups)
1 tablespoon extra-virgin olive oil
2 cups 2% plain Greek yogurt
½ cup chopped walnuts
4 teaspoons honey

Directions
1.   **Preparing the Ingredients**

Place a large, rimmed baking sheet in the oven. Preheat the oven to 450°F with the pan inside. Wash the grapes and remove from the stems. Dry on a clean kitchen towel, and put in a bowl. Drizzle with the oil, and toss to coat.
2.   **Cooking**.
Carefully remove the hot pan from the oven, and pour the grapes onto the pan. Bake for 20 to 23 minutes, until slightly shriveled, stirring once halfway through. Remove the baking sheet from the oven and cool on a wire rack for 5 minutes. While the grapes are cooling, assemble the parfaits by spooning the yogurt into four bowls or tall glasses. Top each bowl or glass with 2 tablespoons of walnuts and 1 teaspoon of honey. When the grapes are slightly cooled, top each parfait with a quarter of the grapes. Scrape any accumulated sweet grape juice onto the parfaits and serve.

Chocolate Banana Smoothie

PREP: 5 MINUTES • COOK TIME: NONE • TOTAL: 5 MINUTES• SERVES: 2

Ingredients
2 bananas, peeled
1 cup unsweetened almond milk, or skim milk
1 cup crushed ice
3 tablespoons unsweetened cocoa powder
3 tablespoons honey

Directions
1.   **Preparing the Ingredients**
Smoothies are great for breakfast on the go because they are quick, fill you up, and provide lasting energy throughout the morning. You can refrigerate leftovers and reblend the next day for about 30 seconds on high speed. In a blender, combine the bananas, almond milk, ice, cocoa powder, and honey. Blend until smooth.

Cherry Almond Baked Oatmeal Cups

PREP: 10 MINUTES, PLUS 10 MINUTES TO COOL • COOK TIME: 35-45 MINUTES • TOTAL: 1 HOUR• SERVES: 6

Ingredients
½ cup gluten-free old-fashioned oats
2 tablespoons sliced almonds
Pinch salt
¾ cup milk
½ teaspoon almond extract
½ teaspoon vanilla
1 egg, beaten
2 tablespoons maple syrup
1 cup frozen cherries, thawed
Ricotta cheese (optional, for topping)
Greek yogurt (optional, for topping)

Directions
1.   **Preparing the Ingredients**
Preheat the oven to 350°F and set the rack to the middle position. Oil two 8-ounce ramekins and place them on a baking sheet. In a medium bowl, combine

all of the ingredients and mix well. Spoon half of the mixture into each ramekin.

2. Cooking

Bake for 35 to 45 minutes, or until the oats are set and a knife inserted into the middle comes out clean. They will be soft but should not be runny.

Let the baked oats cool for 5 to 10 minutes. Top with ricotta cheese or plain Greek yogurt, if desired.

Mashed Chickpea, Feta, And Avocado Toast

PREP: 10 MINUTES • COOK TIME: 15 MINUTES • TOTAL: 25 MINUTES• SERVES: 4

Ingredients

1 (15-ounce) can chickpeas, drained and rinsed
1 avocado, pitted
½ cup diced feta cheese (about 2 ounces)
2 teaspoons freshly squeezed lemon juice or 1 tablespoon orange juice
½ teaspoon freshly ground black pepper
4 pieces multigrain toast
2 teaspoons honey

Directions

1. Preparing the Ingredients

Put the chickpeas in a large bowl. Scoop the avocado flesh into the bowl.

With a potato masher or large fork, mash the ingredients together until the mix has a spreadable consistency. It doesn't need to be totally smooth. Add the feta, lemon juice, and pepper, and mix well.

Evenly divide the mash onto the four pieces of toast and spread with a knife. Drizzle with honey and serve.

Egg In A "Pepper Hole" With Avocado

PREP: 15 MINUTES • COOK TIME: 5 MINUTES • TOTAL: 20 MINUTES• SERVES: 4

Ingredients

4 bell peppers, any color
1 tablespoon extra-virgin olive oil
8 large eggs
¾ teaspoon kosher salt, divided
¼ teaspoon freshly ground black pepper, divided
1 avocado, peeled, pitted, and diced
¼ cup red onion, diced
¼ cup fresh basil, chopped
Juice of ½ lime

Directions

1. Preparing the Ingredients

Stem and seed the bell peppers. Cut 2 (2-inch-thick) rings from each pepper. Chop the remaining bell pepper into small dice, and set aside.

2. Cooking

Heat the olive oil in a large skillet over medium heat. Add 4 bell pepper rings, then crack 1 egg in the middle of each ring. Season with ¼ teaspoon of the salt and ⅛ teaspoon of the black pepper. Cook until the egg whites are mostly set but the yolks are still runny, 2 to 3 minutes. Gently flip and cook 1 additional minute for over easy. Move the egg–bell pepper rings to a platter or onto plates, and repeat with the remaining 4 bell pepper rings.

In a medium bowl, combine the avocado, onion, basil, lime juice, reserved diced bell pepper, the remaining ¼ teaspoon kosher salt, and the remaining ⅛ teaspoon black pepper. Divide among the 4 plates.

Fruit Smoothie

PREP: 5 MINUTES • COOK TIME: NONE • TOTAL: 5 MINUTES• SERVES: 2

Ingredients

2 cups blueberries (or any fresh or frozen fruit, cut into pieces if the fruit is large)
2 cups unsweetened almond milk
1 cup crushed ice
½ teaspoon ground ginger (or other dried ground spice such as turmeric, cinnamon, or nutmeg)

Directions

1. Preparing the Ingredients

In a blender, combine the blueberries, almond milk, ice, and ginger. Blend until smooth.

Some flavor combinations to try: ginger and blueberry, honeydew melon and turmeric, mango and nutmeg, or mixed berries and cinnamon. Have fun experimenting!

The great thing about fruit smoothies is how easy it is to customize them using-seasonal produce. Because fruit is naturally sweet, you don't need to add any additional sweetener here. If using seasonal fruits, opt for fresh. In the absence of seasonal fruits, use frozen fruits.

Individual Baked Egg Casseroles

PREP: 10 MINUTES • COOK TIME: 30 MINUTES • TOTAL: 40 MINUTES• SERVES: 2

Ingredients

1 slice whole-grain bread
4 large eggs, beaten
3 tablespoons milk
¼ teaspoon salt
½ teaspoon onion powder
¼ teaspoon garlic powder
Pinch freshly ground black pepper
¾ cup chopped vegetables (any kind you like)

Directions

1. Preparing the Ingredients

Heat the oven to 375°F and set the rack to the middle position. Oil two 8-ounce ramekins and place them on a baking sheet. Tear the bread into pieces and line each ramekin with ½ of a slice. Mix the eggs, milk, salt, onion powder, garlic powder, pepper, and vegetables in a medium bowl. Pour half of the egg mixture into each ramekin.

2. Cooking

Bake for 30 minutes, or until the eggs are set.

Quickie Honey Nut Granola

PREP: 10 MINUTES • COOK TIME: 20 MINUTES • TOTAL: 30 MINUTES• SERVES: 6

Ingredients

2½ cups regular rolled oats
⅓ cup coarsely chopped almonds
⅛ teaspoon kosher or sea salt
½ teaspoon ground cinnamon
½ cup chopped dried apricots
2 tablespoons ground flaxseed
¼ cup honey
¼ cup extra-virgin olive oil
2 teaspoons vanilla extract
Directions
1.   Preparing the Ingredients
Preheat the oven to 325°F. Line a large, rimmed baking sheet with parchment paper.
2.   Cooking
n a large skillet, combine the oats, almonds, salt, and cinnamon. Turn the heat to medium-high and cook, stirring often, to toast, about 6 minutes. While the oat mixture is toasting, in a microwave-safe bowl, combine the apricots, flaxseed, honey, and oil. Microwave on high for about 1 minute, or until very hot and just beginning to bubble. (Or heat these ingredients in a small saucepan over medium heat for about 3 minutes.)
Stir the vanilla into the honey mixture, then pour it over the oat mixture in the skillet. Stir well.
Spread out the granola on the prepared baking sheet. Bake for 15 minutes, until lightly browned. Remove from the oven and cool completely. Break the granola into small pieces, and store in an airtight container in the refrigerator for up to 2 weeks.

Polenta With Sautéed Chard And Fried Eggs

PREP: 5 MINUTES • COOK TIME: 20 MINUTES • TOTAL: 25 MINUTES• SERVES: 4
Ingredients
2½ cups water
½ teaspoon kosher salt
¾ cups whole-grain cornmeal
¼ teaspoon freshly ground black pepper
2 tablespoons grated Parmesan cheese
1 tablespoon extra-virgin olive oil
1 bunch (about 6 ounces) Swiss chard, leaves and stems chopped and separated
2 garlic cloves, sliced
¼ teaspoon kosher salt
⅛ teaspoon freshly ground black pepper
Lemon juice (optional)
1 tablespoon extra-virgin olive oil
4 large eggs
Directions
1.   Preparing the Ingredients
Bring the water and salt to a boil in a medium saucepan over high heat. Slowly add the cornmeal, whisking constantly. Decrease the heat to low, cover, and cook for 10 to 15 minutes, stirring often to avoid lumps. Stir in the pepper and Parmesan, and divide among 4 bowls.
2.   Cooking

Heat the oil in a large skillet over medium heat. Add the chard stems, garlic, salt, and pepper; sauté for 2 minutes. Add the chard leaves and cook until wilted, about 3 to 5 minutes. Add a spritz of lemon juice (if desired), toss together, and divide evenly on top of the polenta.
Heat the oil in the same large skillet over medium-high heat. Crack each egg into the skillet, taking care not to crowd the skillet and leaving space between the eggs. Cook until the whites are set and golden around the edges, about 2 to 3 minutes.
Serve sunny-side up or flip the eggs over carefully and cook 1 minute longer for over easy. Place one egg on top of the polenta and chard in each bowl.

Berry And Yogurt Parfait

PREP: 5 MINUTES • COOK TIME: NONE • TOTAL: 5 MINUTES• SERVES: 2
Ingredients
1 cup raspberries
1½ cups unsweetened nonfat plain Greek yogurt
1 cup blackberries
¼ cup chopped walnuts
Directions
Preparing the Ingredients
In 2 bowls, layer the raspberries, yogurt, and blackberries. Sprinkle with the walnuts.
You can use any berries you like here, but the raspberries and blackberries in this recipe add a nice variety of flavors, and they don't require any chopping. These parfaits are especially good in the summer when berries are in season. Feel free to substitute any chopped fresh fruit.

Overnight Pomegranate Muesli

PREP: 10 MINUTES, PLUS OVERNIGHT TO CHILL • COOK TIME: 30 MINUTES • TOTAL: 40 MINUTES• SERVES: 2
Ingredients
½ cup gluten-free old-fashioned oats
¼ cup shelled pistachios
3 tablespoons pumpkin seeds
2 tablespoons chia seeds
¾ cup milk
½ cup plain Greek yogurt
2 to 3 teaspoons maple syrup (optional)
½ cup pomegranate arils
Directions
Preparing the Ingredients
In a medium bowl, mix together the oats, pistachios, pumpkin seeds, chia seeds, milk, yogurt, and maple syrup, if using.
Divide the mixture between two 12-ounce mason jars or another type of container with a lid.
Top each with ¼ cup of pomegranate arils.
Cover each jar or container and store in the refrigerator overnight or up to 4 days.
Serve cold, with additional milk if desired.

Breakfast Polenta

PREP: 5 MINUTES • COOK TIME: 10 MINUTES • TOTAL: 15 MINUTES• SERVES: 6

Ingredients

2 (18-ounce) tubes plain polenta

2¼ to 2½ cups 2% milk, divided

2 oranges, peeled and chopped

½ cup chopped pecans

¼ cup 2% plain Greek yogurt

8 teaspoons honey

Directions

Preparing the Ingredients

1. Slice the polenta into rounds and place in a microwave-safe bowl. Heat in the microwave on high for 45 seconds.

Transfer the polenta to a large pot, and mash it with a potato masher or fork until coarsely mashed. Place the pot on the stove over medium heat.

2. In a medium, microwave-safe bowl, heat the milk in the microwave on high for 1 minute. Pour 2 cups of the warmed milk into the pot with the polenta, and stir with a whisk. Continue to stir and mash with the whisk, adding the remaining milk a few tablespoons at a time, until the polenta is fairly smooth and heated through, about 5 minutes. Remove from the stove.

3. Divide the polenta among four serving bowls. Top each bowl with one-quarter of the oranges, 2 tablespoons of pecans, 1 tablespoon of yogurt, and 2 teaspoons of honey before serving.

Smoked Salmon Egg Scramble With Dill And Chives

PREP: 5 MINUTES • COOK TIME: 5 MINUTES • TOTAL: 10 MINUTES • SERVES: 2

Ingredients

4 large eggs

1 tablespoon milk

1 tablespoon fresh chives, minced

1 tablespoon fresh dill, minced

¼ teaspoon kosher salt

⅛ teaspoon freshly ground black pepper

2 teaspoons extra-virgin olive oil

2 ounces smoked salmon, thinly sliced

Directions

1. **Preparing the Ingredients**

In a large bowl, whisk together the eggs, milk, chives, dill, salt, and pepper.

2. **Cooking**

Heat the olive oil in a medium skillet or sauté pan over medium heat. Add the egg mixture and cook for about 3 minutes, stirring occasionally.

Add the salmon and cook until the eggs are set but moist, about 1 minute.

Yogurt With Blueberries, Honey, And Mint

PREP: 5 MINUTES • COOK TIME: NONE• TOTAL: 5 MINUTES• SERVES: 2

Ingredients

2 cups unsweetened nonfat plain Greek yogurt

1 cup blueberries

3 tablespoons honey

2 tablespoons fresh mint leaves, chopped

Directions

Preparing the Ingredients

Apportion the yogurt between 2 small bowls. Top with the blueberries, honey, and mint.

Mediterranean Breakfast Pizza

PREP: 5 MINUTES • COOK TIME: 15 MINUTES • TOTAL: 20 MINUTES• SERVES: 2

Ingredients

2 (6- to 8-inch-long) pieces of whole-wheat naan bread

2 tablespoons prepared pesto

1 medium tomato, sliced

2 large eggs

Directions

1. **Preparing the Ingredients**

Heat a large nonstick skillet over medium-high heat. Place the naan bread in the skillet and let it warm for about 2 minutes on each side. The bread should be softened and just starting to turn golden. Spread 1 tablespoon of the pesto on one side of each slice. Top the pesto with tomato slices to cover. Remove the pizzas from the pan and place each one on its own plate.

Crack the eggs into the pan, keeping them separated, and cook until the whites are no longer translucent and the yolk is cooked to desired doneness. With a spatula, spoon one egg onto each pizza.

SNACKS AND SIDES

White Bean Harissa Dip

PREP TIME: 10 MINUTES / COOK TIME: 1 HOUR / TOTAL: 1 HOUR 10 MINUTES / MAKES 1½ CUPS

Ingredients

1 whole head of garlic
½ cup olive oil, divided
1 (15-ounce) can cannellini beans, drained and rinsed
1 teaspoon salt
1 teaspoon harissa paste (or more to taste)

Directions

1.   Preparing the Ingredients

Preheat the oven to 350°F.

Cut about ½ inch off the top of a whole head of garlic and lightly wrap it in foil. Drizzle 1 to 2 teaspoons of olive oil over the top of the cut side.

2.   Cooking

Place it in an oven-safe dish and roast it in the oven for about 1 hour or until the cloves are soft and tender.

Remove the garlic from the oven and let it cool. The garlic can be roasted up to 2 days ahead of time.

Remove the garlic cloves from their skin and place them in the bowl of a food processor along with the beans, salt, and harissa. Purée, drizzling in as much olive oil as needed until the beans are smooth. If the dip seems too stiff, add additional olive oil to loosen the dip. Taste the dip and add additional salt, harissa, or oil as needed.

Store in the refrigerator for up to a week. Portion out ¼ cup of dip and serve with a mixture of raw vegetables and mini pita breads.

Mediterranean Fruit, Veggie, and Cheese Board

PREP TIME: 15 MINUTES / COOK TIME: 1 HOUR / TOTAL: 1 HOUR PLUS 15 MINUTES / SERVES 4

Ingredients

2 cups sliced fruits, such as apples, pears, plums, or peaches
2 cups finger-food fruits, such as berries, cherries, grapes, or figs
2 cups raw vegetables cut into sticks, such as carrots, celery, broccoli, cauliflower, or whole cherry tomatoes
1 cup cured, canned, or jarred vegetables, such as roasted peppers or artichoke hearts, or ½ cup olives
1 cup cubed cheese, such as goat cheese, Gorgonzola, feta, Manchego, or Asiago (about 4 ounces)

Directions

Preparing the Ingredients

1.   Wash all the fresh produce and cut into slices or bite-size pieces, as described in the ingredients list.

2.   Arrange all the ingredients on a wooden board or serving tray. Include small spoons for items like the berries and olives, and a fork or knife for the cheeses. Serve with small plates and napkins.

Summer Squash Ribbons with Lemon and Ricotta

PREP TIME: 20 MINUTES / COOK TIME: 1 HOUR / TOTAL: 1 HOUR 20 MINUTES / MAKES ½ CUPS

Ingredients

2 medium zucchini or yellow squash
½ cup ricotta cheese
2 tablespoons fresh mint, chopped, plus additional mint leaves for garnish
2 tablespoons fresh parsley, chopped
Zest of ½ lemon
2 teaspoons lemon juice
½ teaspoon kosher salt
¼ teaspoon freshly ground black pepper
1 tablespoon extra-virgin olive oil

Directions

Preparing the Ingredients

1.   Using a vegetable peeler, make ribbons by peeling the summer squash lengthwise.
The squash ribbons will resemble the wide pasta, pappardelle.

2.   In a medium bowl, combine the ricotta cheese, mint, parsley, lemon zest, lemon juice, salt, and black pepper. Place mounds of the squash ribbons evenly on 4 plates then dollop the ricotta mixture on top. Drizzle with the olive oil and garnish with the mint leaves.

HUMMUS

PREP TIME: 10 MINUTES / COOK TIME: 30 MINUTES/ TOTAL: 40 MINUTES / MAKES 1-4 OUNCE

Ingredients

1 (14-ounce) can chickpeas, drained
3 garlic cloves, minced
2 tablespoons tahini
2 tablespoons extra-virgin olive oil
Juice of 1 lemon
Zest of 1 lemon
½ teaspoon sea salt
Pinch cayenne pepper
2 tablespoons chopped fresh Italian parsley leaves

Directions

Preparing the Ingredients

1.   In a blender, combine the chickpeas, garlic, tahini, olive oil, lemon juice and zest, sea salt and cayenne. Blend for about 60 seconds until smooth. Garnish with parsley and serve.

Mediterranean Trail Mix

PREP TIME: 10 MINUTES / COOK TIME: 10 MINUTES/ TOTAL: 20 MINUTES / MAKES 4 CUPS

Ingredients

1 tablespoon olive oil
1 tablespoon maple syrup

1 teaspoon vanilla
½ teaspoon cardamom
½ teaspoon allspice
2 cups mixed, unsalted nuts
¼ cup unsalted pumpkin or sunflower seeds
½ cup dried apricots, diced or thin sliced
½ cup dried figs, diced or thinly sliced
Pinch salt

Directions

1. **Preparing the Ingredients.** Combine the olive oil, maple syrup, vanilla, cardamom, and allspice in a large sauté pan over medium heat. Stir to combine. Add the nuts and seeds and stir well to coat. Let the nuts and seeds toast for about 10 minutes, stirring frequently. Remove from the heat, and add the dried apricots and figs. Stir everything well and season with salt. Store in an airtight container. Nuts are a great thing to buy in bulk. As long as you store them in airtight containers, they'll last for a few months. Look for raw nuts that don't have added salt or sugar. That way you can toast them and flavor them in any way you like.

Quick Toasted Almonds

PREP TIME: 10 MINUTES / COOK TIME: 30 MINUTES/ MAKES 2 CUPS

Ingredients

1 tablespoon extra-virgin olive oil
2 cups skin-on raw whole almonds
1 teaspoon salt
¼ teaspoon pepper

Directions

1. **Preparing the Ingredients**

Heat oil in 12-inch nonstick skillet over medium-high heat until just shimmering. Add almonds, salt, and pepper and reduce heat to medium-low. Cook, stirring often, until almonds are fragrant and their color deepens slightly, about 8 minutes. Transfer almonds to paper towel–lined plate and let cool before serving. (Almonds can be stored at room temperature for up to 5 days.)

Lemony Garlic Hummus

PREP TIME: 10 MINUTES / COOK TIME: NONE / SERVES 6

Ingredients

1 (15-ounce) can chickpeas
Drained
Liquid reserved
3 tablespoons freshly squeezed lemon juice (from about 1 large lemon)
2 tablespoons peanut butter
3 tablespoons extra-virgin olive oil, divided
2 garlic cloves
¼ teaspoon kosher or sea salt (optional)
Raw veggies or whole-grain crackers, for serving (optional)

Directions

1. **Preparing the Ingredients**

In the bowl of a food processor, combine the chickpeas and 2 tablespoons of the reserved chickpea liquid with the lemon juice, peanut butter, 2 tablespoons of oil, and the garlic. Process the mixture for 1 minute. Scrape down the sides of the bowl with a rubber spatula. Process for 1 more minute, or until smooth.

Put in a serving bowl, drizzle with the remaining 1 tablespoon of olive oil, sprinkle with the salt, if using, and serve with veggies or crackers, if desired.

The key to light, airy hummus is to add some chickpea liquid, also known as aquafaba. While we usually recommend draining and rinsing canned beans to remove more sodium, for this recipe, save that liquid gold to make your hummus beyond delicious.

Sautéed Kale with Tomato and Garlic

PREP TIME: 10 MINUTES / COOK TIME: 5 MINUTES/ MAKES 14.5 OUNCE/ SERVES 4

Ingredients

1 tablespoon extra-virgin olive oil
4 garlic cloves, sliced
¼ teaspoon red pepper flakes
2 bunches kale, stemmed and chopped or torn into pieces
1 (14.5-ounce) can no-salt-added diced tomatoes
½ teaspoon kosher salt

Directions

1. **Preparing the Ingredients**

Heat the olive oil in a wok or large skillet over medium-high heat. Add the garlic and red pepper flakes, and sauté until fragrant, about 30 seconds. Add the kale and sauté, about 3 to 5 minutes, until the kale shrinks down a bit. Add the tomatoes and the salt, stir together, and cook for 3 to 5 minutes, or until the liquid reduces and the kale cooks down further and becomes tender. Adding garlic and red pepper flakes to the oil first allows the flavors to permeate the oil, creating more flavor for the overall dish. If this makes the dish too spicy for your palate, eliminate the red pepper flakes or add them in step 2 with the salt and tomatoes.

Baba Ganoush

PREP TIME: 10 MINUTES / COOK TIME: 15 MINUTES/ MAKES ½ CUP

Ingredients

1 eggplant, peeled and sliced
¼ cup tahini
½ teaspoon sea salt
Juice of 1 lemon
¼ teaspoon ground cumin
⅛ teaspoon freshly ground black pepper
2 tablespoons extra-virgin olive oil
2 tablespoons sunflower seeds (optional)
2 tablespoons fresh Italian parsley leaves (optional)

Directions

1. **Preparing the Ingredients**

Preheat the oven to 350°F. On a baking sheet, spread the eggplant slices in an even layer.

2.   **Cooking**

Bake for about 15 minutes until soft. Cool slightly and roughly chop the eggplant. In a blender, blend the eggplant with the tahini, sea salt, lemon juice, cumin, and pepper for about 30 seconds. Transfer to a serving dish. Drizzle with the olive oil and sprinkle with the sunflower seeds and parsley (if using) before serving. You can also make Baba Ganoush with zucchini in place of the eggplant. Halve 4 zucchini lengthwise (no need to peel!) and cook in a 350°F oven for about 10 minutes until soft. Continue with the recipe as directed.

Seared Halloumi with Pesto and Tomato

PREP TIME: 2 MINUTES / COOK TIME: 5 MINUTES/ MAKES ½ CUPS

Ingredients

3 ounces Halloumi cheese, cut crosswise into 2 thinner, rectangular pieces
2 teaspoons prepared pesto sauce, plus additional for drizzling if desired
1 medium tomato, sliced

Directions

1.   **Preparing the Ingredients**

Heat a nonstick skillet over medium-high heat and place the slices of Halloumi in the hot pan. After about 2 minutes, check to see if the cheese is golden on the bottom. If it is, flip the slices, top each with 1 teaspoon of pesto, and cook for another 2 minutes, or until the second side is golden. Serve with slices of tomato and a drizzle of pesto, if desired, on the side. Because Halloumi is a fairly salty cheese, no additional salt is needed in this dish.

Romesco Dip

PREP TIME: 10 MINUTES / COOK TIME: NONE/ MAKES 12 OUNCE / SERVES 10

Ingredients

1 (12-ounce) jar roasted red peppers, drained
1 (14.5-ounce) can diced tomatoes, undrained
½ cup dry-roasted almonds
2 garlic cloves
2 teaspoons red wine vinegar
1 teaspoon smoked paprika or ½ teaspoon cayenne pepper
¼ teaspoon kosher or sea salt
¼ teaspoon freshly ground black pepper
¼ cup extra-virgin olive oil
⅔ cup torn, day-old bread or toast (about 2 slices)
Assortment of sliced raw vegetables such as carrots, celery, cucumber, green beans, and bell peppers, for serving

Directions

1.   **Preparing the Ingredients**

In a high-powered blender or food processor, combine the roasted peppers, tomatoes and their juices, almonds, garlic, vinegar, smoked paprika, salt, and pepper. Begin puréeing the ingredients on medium speed, and slowly drizzle in the oil with the blender running. Continue to purée until the dip is thoroughly mixed. Add the bread and purée.
Serve with raw vegetables for dipping, or store in a jar with a lid for up to one week in the refrigerator.

Roasted Broccoli with Tahini Yogurt Sauce

PREP TIME: 15 MINUTES / COOK TIME: 30 MINUTES/ MAKES ½ CUPS / SERVES 4

Ingredients

1½ to 2 pounds broccoli, stalk trimmed and cut into slices, head cut into florets
1 lemon, sliced into ¼-inch-thick rounds
3 tablespoons extra-virgin olive oil
½ teaspoon kosher salt
¼ teaspoon freshly ground black pepper
½ cup plain Greek yogurt
2 tablespoons tahini
1 tablespoon lemon juice
¼ teaspoon kosher salt
1 teaspoon sesame seeds, for garnish (optional)

Directions

1.   **Preparing the Ingredients**

Preheat the oven to 425°F. Line a baking sheet with parchment paper or foil.
In a large bowl, gently toss the broccoli, lemon slices, olive oil, salt, and black pepper to combine. Arrange the broccoli in a single layer on the prepared baking sheet.

2.   **Cooking**

Roast 15 minutes, stir, and roast another 15 minutes, until golden brown. In a medium bowl, combine the yogurt, tahini, lemon juice, and salt; mix well. Spread the tahini yogurt sauce on a platter or large plate and top with the broccoli and lemon slices. Garnish with the sesame seeds (if desired). Lining your baking sheet with parchment paper or foil makes cleanup a breeze. Simply crumple up and throw away with no need to scrub brown bits off the pan.

Spiced Almonds

PREP TIME: 10 MINUTES / COOK TIME: 7 MINUTES/ MAKES ½ CUPS / SERVES 8

Ingredients

2 cups raw unsalted almonds
1 tablespoon extra-virgin olive oil
1 teaspoon ground cumin
½ teaspoon garlic powder
½ teaspoon sea salt
⅛ teaspoon cayenne pepper

Directions

1.   **Preparing the Ingredients**

In a large nonstick skillet over medium-high heat, cook the almonds for about 3 minutes, shaking the pan constantly, until the almonds become fragrant. Transfer to a bowl and set aside. In the same skillet over medium-high heat, heat the olive oil until it shimmers. Add the cumin, garlic powder, sea salt, and cayenne. Cook for 30 to 60 seconds, until the spices become fragrant. Add the almonds to the skillet. Cook for about 3 minutes more, stirring, until the spices coat the almonds. Let cool before serving.

Stuffed Cucumber Cups

PREP TIME: 5 MINUTES / COOK TIME: 30 MINUTES/ MAKES 8 OUNCES / SERVES 2

Ingredients

1 medium cucumber (about 8 ounces, 8 to 9 inches long)
½ cup hummus (any flavor) or white bean dip
4 or 5 cherry tomatoes, sliced in half
2 tablespoons fresh basil, minced

Directions

1.   Preparing the Ingredients

Slice the ends off the cucumber (about ½ inch from each side) and slice the cucumber into 1-inch pieces. With a paring knife or a spoon, scoop most of the seeds from the inside of each cucumber piece to make a cup, being careful to not cut all the way through. Fill each cucumber cup with about 1 tablespoon of hummus or bean dip.

Top each with a cherry tomato half and a sprinkle of fresh minced basil. Experiment with different toppings such as chopped olives, sun-dried tomatoes, or feta cheese instead of the cherry tomatoes and basil.

Eggplant Relish Spread

PREP TIME: 10 MINUTES / COOK TIME: 20 MINUTES/ MAKES ONE POT / SERVES 6

Ingredients

2 tablespoons extra-virgin olive oil
1 cup finely chopped onion (about ½ medium onion)
1 garlic clove, minced (about ½ teaspoon)
1 large globe eggplant, cut into ½-inch cubes (about 5 cups)
¼ teaspoon kosher or sea salt
1 (12-ounce) jar roasted red peppers, chopped
1½ cups chopped fresh tomatoes
½ cup balsamic or red wine vinegar
½ cup capers or chopped olives

Directions

1.   Preparing the Ingredients

In a large skillet over medium heat, heat the oil. Add the onion and cook for 4 minutes, stirring occasionally. Add the garlic and cook for 1 minute, stirring often. Turn up the heat to medium-high, and add the eggplant and salt. Cook for 5 minutes, stirring occasionally. Add the peppers, tomatoes, and vinegar, stir, and cover. Cook for 10 minutes, stirring every minute or so to prevent everything from sticking. If it looks like it's starting to stick and burn, turn down the heat to medium and add 1 tablespoon of water. Remove from the heat, stir in the capers, and let sit for a few minutes to let the liquid absorb. Stir and serve, or store in a covered jar in the refrigerator for up to 10 days. It tastes even better the day after you make it!

SOUPS AND SALADS

Hearty Italian Turkey Vegetable Soup

PREP TIME: 30 MINUTES / COOK TIME: 1 HOUR 10 MINUTES / SERVES 2 WITH 2 SERVINGS FOR LEFTOVERS

Ingredients

1 tablespoon olive oil
½ pound lean ground turkey
1 celery stalk, diced (about ¼ cup)
2 medium carrots, diced (about ¾ cup)
1 small onion, diced (about 1 cup)
1 small fennel bulb, diced (about 1 cup)
1 garlic clove, minced
1 large leaf lacinato (dinosaur) kale, stemmed and chopped
2½ cups low-sodium tomato juice
2 cups low-sodium chicken stock
1 (15-ounce) can kidney beans, drained and rinsed
¾ teaspoon fennel seeds
¼ teaspoon red pepper flakes (optional)
¾ cup small shell pasta
2 tablespoons fresh basil, thinly sliced (about 4 basil leaves)
Salt

Directions

1.   **Preparing the Ingredients**
Heat the olive oil in a stockpot over medium-high heat. Add the turkey and sauté for 10 minutes, or until it's no longer pink.
2.   **Cooking**
Add the celery, carrots, onion, fennel, garlic, and kale and sauté for about 10 minutes. Add the tomato juice, chicken stock, kidney beans, fennel seeds, and red pepper flakes and bring the soup to a boil. Reduce the heat, cover the pot, and let the soup simmer for 40 minutes, or until the carrots are softened. Add the pasta and cook for another 10 minutes, or until al dente. Add the basil, and season with salt to taste—start with about ½ teaspoon.

Pistachio Parmesan Kale-Arugula Salad

PREP TIME: 20 MINUTES / COOK TIME: 10 MINUTES/ SERVES 6

Ingredients

6 cups raw kale, center ribs removed and discarded, leaves coarsely chopped
¼ cup extra-virgin olive oil
2 tablespoons freshly squeezed lemon juice (from about 1 small lemon)
½ teaspoon smoked paprika
2 cups arugula
⅓ cup unsalted shelled pistachios
6 tablespoons grated Parmesan or Pecorino Romano cheese

Directions

1.   **Preparing the Ingredients**
In a large salad bowl, combine the kale, oil, lemon juice, and smoked paprika. With your hands, gently massage the leaves for about 15 seconds or so, until all are thoroughly coated. Let the kale sit for 10 minutes.

When you're ready to serve, gently mix in the arugula and pistachios. Divide the salad among six serving bowls, sprinkle 1 tablespoon of grated cheese over each, and serve.

Pistachio Quinoa Salad with Pomegranate Citrus Vinaigrette

PREP TIME: 15 MINUTES / COOK TIME: 15 MINUTES/ SERVES 6

Ingredients

1½ cups water
1 cup quinoa
¼ teaspoon kosher salt
1 cup extra-virgin olive oil
½ cup pomegranate juice
½ cup freshly squeezed orange juice
1 small shallot, minced
1 teaspoon pure maple syrup
1 teaspoon za'atar
½ teaspoon ground sumac
½ teaspoon kosher salt
¼ teaspoon freshly ground black pepper
3 cups baby spinach
½ cup fresh parsley, coarsely chopped
½ cup fresh mint, coarsely chopped
Approximately ¾ cup pomegranate seeds, or 2 pomegranates
¼ cup pistachios, shelled and toasted
¼ cup crumbled blue cheese

Directions

1.   **Preparing the Ingredients**
Bring the water, quinoa, and salt to a boil in a small saucepan. Reduce the heat and cover; simmer for 10 to 12 minutes. Fluff with a fork. In a medium bowl, whisk together the olive oil, pomegranate juice, orange juice, shallot, maple syrup, za'atar, sumac, salt, and black pepper. In a large bowl, add about ½ cup of dressing.

Store the remaining dressing in a glass jar or airtight container and refrigerate.

The dressing can be kept up to 2 weeks.

Let the chilled dressing reach room temperature before using. Combine the spinach, parsley, and mint in the bowl with the dressing and toss gently together. Add the quinoa. Toss gently.

Add the pomegranate seeds. Or, if using whole pomegranates: Cut the pomegranates in half. Fill a large bowl with water and hold the pomegranate half, cut side-down. Using a wooden spoon, hit the back of the pomegranate so the seeds fall into the water. Immerse the pomegranate in the water and gently pull out any remaining seeds.

Repeat with the remaining pomegranate. Skim the white pith off the top of the water. Drain the seeds and add them to the greens. Add the pistachios and cheese and toss gently.

You can use any citrus juice you like for the dressing. Try lemon, lime, or grapefruit in place of orange.

Greek Salad

PREP TIME: 10 MINUTES / COOK TIME: NONE/ SERVES 4

Ingredients

1 head romaine lettuce, torn
½ cup black olives, pitted and chopped
1 red onion, thinly sliced
1 tomato, chopped
1 cucumber, chopped
½ cup crumbled feta cheese
2 tablespoons extra-virgin olive oil
2 tablespoons red wine vinegar
Juice of 1 lemon
1 tablespoon dried oregano (or 2 tablespoons chopped fresh oregano leaves)
3 garlic cloves, minced
½ teaspoon Dijon mustard
½ teaspoon sea salt
¼ teaspoon freshly ground black pepper

Directions

1. **Preparing the Ingredients**

In a large bowl, mix the lettuce, olives, red onion, tomato, cucumber, and feta.

To make the dressing: In a small bowl, whisk the olive oil, vinegar, lemon juice, oregano, garlic, mustard, sea salt, and pepper.

Just before serving, toss the salad with the dressing. Add 4 chopped hardboiled eggs to make this a hearty protein-filled meal.

Creamy Tomato Hummus Soup

PREP TIME: 10 MINUTES / COOK TIME: 10 MINUTES / SERVES 2 WITH 2 SERVINGS FOR LEFTOVERS

Ingredients

1 (14.5-ounce) can crushed tomatoes with basil
1 cup roasted red pepper hummus
2 cups low-sodium chicken stock
Salt
¼ cup fresh basil leaves, thinly sliced (optional, for garnish)
Garlic croutons (optional, for garnish)

Directions

Preparing the Ingredients

1. Combine the canned tomatoes, hummus, and chicken stock in a blender and blend until smooth. Pour the mixture into a saucepan and bring it to a boil.

Season with salt and fresh basil if desired. Serve with garlic croutons as a garnish, if desired.

2. To make this a heartier soup, add shredded chicken and precooked brown rice or barley.

Easy Italian Orange and Celery Salad

PREP TIME: 15 MINUTES / COOK TIME: NONE/ SERVES 6

Ingredients

3 celery stalks, including leaves, sliced diagonally into ½-inch slices
2 large oranges, peeled and sliced into rounds
½ cup green olives (or any variety)
¼ cup sliced red onion (about ¼ onion)
1 tablespoon extra-virgin olive oil
1 tablespoon olive brine
1 tablespoon freshly squeezed lemon or orange juice (from ½ small lemon or 1 orange round)
¼ teaspoon kosher or sea salt
¼ teaspoon freshly ground black pepper

Directions

Preparing the Ingredients

1. Place the celery, oranges, olives, and onion on a large serving platter or in a shallow, wide bowl.

2. In a small bowl, whisk together the oil, olive brine, and lemon juice. Pour over the salad, sprinkle with salt and pepper, and serve.

3. Instead of the orange rounds in this salad, you can swap in peeled and sectioned clementines or canned mandarin oranges in juice that have been drained.

Cauliflower Tabbouleh Salad

PREP TIME: 15 MINUTES / COOK TIME: 0 MINUTES / SERVES 4

Ingredients

¼ cup extra-virgin olive oil
¼ cup lemon juice
Zest of 1 lemon
¾ teaspoon kosher salt
½ teaspoon ground turmeric
¼ teaspoon ground coriander
¼ teaspoon ground cumin
¼ teaspoon black pepper
⅛ teaspoon ground cinnamon
1 pound riced cauliflower
1 English cucumber, diced
12 cherry tomatoes, halved
1 cup fresh parsley, chopped
½ cup fresh mint, chopped

Directions

Preparing the Ingredients

1. In a large bowl, whisk together the olive oil, lemon juice, lemon zest, salt, turmeric, coriander, cumin, black pepper, and cinnamon.

2. Add the riced cauliflower to the bowl and mix well. Add in the cucumber, tomatoes, parsley, and mint and gently mix together.

Cucumber Salad

PREP TIME: 15 MINUTES / COOK TIME: NONE/ SERVES 4

Ingredients

4 medium cucumbers, chopped or spiralized into spaghetti noodles
1 tomato, chopped

3 scallions, white and green parts, chopped
2 tablespoons extra-virgin olive oil
¼ cup red wine vinegar
2 tablespoons chopped fresh dill
2 garlic cloves, minced
1 teaspoon Dijon mustard
½ teaspoon sea salt
¼ teaspoon freshly ground black pepper

Directions

Preparing the Ingredients

1.   In a large bowl, mix together the cucumber, tomato, and scallions.
In a small bowl, whisk the olive oil, vinegar, dill, garlic, mustard, sea salt, and pepper.
Toss the dressing with the salad just before serving. Cucumbers lend themselves nicely to various flavor profiles. To change things up, omit the tomato and add 3 more scallions.

2.   For the dressing: Whisk 2 tablespoons extra-virgin olive oil, ¼ cup apple cider vinegar, 1 tablespoon grated fresh ginger, 3 minced garlic cloves, 2 tablespoons chopped fresh cilantro leaves, ½ teaspoon sea salt, and ⅛ teaspoon freshly ground black pepper.

Spicy Sausage Lentil Soup

PREP TIME: 30 MINUTES / COOK TIME: 60 MINUTES/ SERVES 2 WITH 2 SERVINGS FOR LEFTOVERS

Ingredients

1 tablespoon olive oil
½ medium onion, diced (about ¾ cup)
2 links (8 ounces) spicy Italian sausage (turkey or pork), removed from casing
2 medium carrots, sliced into coins (about ¾ cup)
1 medium celery stalk, diced (about ¼ cup)
2 garlic cloves, minced
¼ teaspoon red pepper flakes (omit or use less if you prefer less spicy)
½ teaspoon thyme
1 teaspoon oregano
1 bay leaf
3 cups low-sodium chicken stock
1 (28-ounce) can crushed tomatoes
¾ cup brown lentils
1 cup packed baby spinach, sliced
½ teaspoon salt, plus more to taste

Directions

Preparing the Ingredients

1.   Heat the oil in a stockpot over medium-high heat. Add the onion and sausage and sauté, breaking up the sausage into small pieces.
Add the carrots, celery, and garlic, and continue to sauté for about 10 more minutes.
Add the red pepper flakes, thyme, oregano, bay leaf, chicken stock, and tomatoes. Bring the soup to a boil.

2.   Reduce the heat to medium-low and add the lentils. Stir everything well, cover, and let the soup simmer for 45 minutes, or until the lentils and carrots are tender.

Remove the bay leaf. Add the spinach and season with salt—start with ½ teaspoon and add additional salt to taste.

Spanish Style Turkey Meatball Soup (Instant Pot)

PREP TIME: 30 MINUTES / COOK TIME: 30 MINUTES/ SERVES 6 TO 8

Ingredients

1 slice hearty white sandwich bread, torn into quarters
¼ cup whole milk
1 ounce Manchego cheese, grated (½ cup), plus extra for serving
5 tablespoons minced fresh parsley, divided
½ teaspoon table salt
1 pound ground turkey
1 tablespoon extra-virgin olive oil
1 onion, chopped
1 red bell pepper, stemmed, seeded, and cut into ¾-inch pieces
4 garlic cloves, minced
2 teaspoons smoked paprika
½ cup dry white wine
8 cups chicken broth
8 ounces kale, stemmed and chopped

Directions

Preparing the Ingredients

1.   Using fork, mash bread and milk together into paste in large bowl. Stir in Manchego, 3 tablespoons parsley, and salt until combined. Add turkey and knead mixture with your hands until well combined. Pinch off and roll 2-teaspoon-size pieces of mixture into balls and arrange on large plate (you should have about 35 meatballs); set aside.
Using highest sauté function, heat oil in Instant Pot until shimmering. Add onion and bell pepper and cook until softened and lightly browned, 5 to 7 minutes. Stir in garlic and paprika and cook until fragrant, about 30 seconds. Stir in wine, scraping up any browned bits, and cook until almost completely evaporated, about 5 minutes. Stir in broth and kale, then gently submerge meatballs.

2.   Lock lid in place and close pressure release valve. Select high pressure cook function and cook for 3 minutes. Turn off Instant Pot and quick-release pressure. Carefully remove lid, allowing steam to escape away from you.

3.   Stir in remaining 2 tablespoons parsley and season with salt and pepper to taste. Serve, passing extra Manchego separately.

Melon Caprese Salad

PREP TIME: 20 MINUTES / COOK TIME: 0 MINUTES/ SERVES 6

Ingredients

1 cantaloupe, quartered and seeded
½ small seedless watermelon
1 cup grape tomatoes
2 cups fresh mozzarella balls (about 8 ounces)

⅓ cup fresh basil or mint leaves, torn into small pieces
2 tablespoons extra-virgin olive oil
1 tablespoon balsamic vinegar
¼ teaspoon freshly ground black pepper
¼ teaspoon kosher or sea salt

Directions

Preparing the Ingredients

1.   Using a melon baller or a metal, teaspoon-size measuring spoon, scoop balls out of the cantaloupe. You should get about 2½ to 3 cups from one cantaloupe. (If you prefer, cut the melon into bite-size pieces instead of making balls.) Put them in a large colander over a large serving bowl.

2.   Using the same method, ball or cut the watermelon into bite-size pieces; you should get about 2 cups. Put the watermelon balls in the colander with the cantaloupe.

3.   Let the fruit drain for 10 minutes. Pour the juice from the bowl into a container to refrigerate and save for drinking or adding to smoothies. Wipe the bowl dry, and put in the cut fruit.

4.   Add the tomatoes, mozzarella, basil, oil, vinegar, pepper, and salt to the fruit mixture. Gently mix until everything is incorporated and serve.

If you want to make this recipe a day ahead, prepare the salad through step 3. Cover and refrigerate. Before serving, drain the fruit again for about 5 minutes. Add it back into the serving bowl, then toss it with the remaining ingredients.

Caprese Salad

PREP TIME: 15 MINUTES / COOK TIME: NONE / SERVES 4

Ingredients

3 large tomatoes, sliced
4 ounces part-skim mozzarella cheese, cut into ¼-inch-thick slices
¼ cup balsamic vinegar
2 tablespoons extra-virgin olive oil
½ teaspoon sea salt
¼ cup loosely packed basil leaves, torn

Directions

Preparing the Ingredients

1.   On a pretty platter, arrange the tomatoes and cheese slices alternating and overlapping in a row.

Drizzle with the vinegar and olive oil.
Sprinkle with sea salt and basil and serve.

2.   Replace the balsamic vinegar with an equal amount of freshly squeezed lemon juice or red wine vinegar.

Vegetable Fagioli

PREP TIME: 30 MINUTES / COOK TIME: 60 MINUTES / SERVES 2 WITH 2 SERVINGS FOR LEFTOVERS

Ingredients

1 tablespoon olive oil
2 medium carrots, diced (about ¾ cup)

2 medium celery stalks, diced (about ½ cup)
½ medium onion, diced (about ¾ cup)
1 large garlic clove, minced
3 tablespoons tomato paste
4 cups low-sodium vegetable broth
1 cup packed kale, stemmed and chopped
1 (15-ounce) can red kidney beans, drained and rinsed
1 (15-ounce) can cannellini beans, drained and rinsed
½ cup fresh basil, chopped
Salt
Freshly ground black pepper

Directions

Preparing the Ingredients

1.   Heat the olive oil in a stockpot over medium-high heat. Add the carrots, celery, onion, and garlic and sauté for 10 minutes, or until the vegetables start to turn golden.

Stir in the tomato paste and cook for about 30 seconds.

2.   Add the vegetable broth and bring the soup to a boil. Cover, and reduce the heat to low. Cook the soup for 45 minutes, or until the carrots are tender.

3.   Using an immersion blender, purée the soup so that it's partly smooth, but with some chunks of vegetables. If you don't have an immersion blender, scoop out about ⅓ of the soup and blend it in a blender, then add it back to the pot.

Add the kale, beans, and basil. Season with salt and pepper.

Classic Chicken Broth

PREP TIME: 15 MINUTES / COOK TIME: 30 MINUTES/ MAKES: 8 CUPS / SERVES 4

Ingredients

4 pounds chicken backs and wings
14 cups water
1 onion, chopped
2 bay leaves
2 teaspoons salt

Directions

1.   Heat chicken and water in large stockpot or Dutch oven over medium-high heat until boiling, skimming off any scum that comes to surface. Reduce heat to low and simmer gently for 3 hours.

Add onion, bay leaves, and salt and continue to simmer for another 2 hours.

2.   Strain broth through fine-mesh strainer into large pot or container, pressing on solids to extract as much liquid as possible. Let broth settle for about 5 minutes, then skim off fat. (Cooled broth can be refrigerated for up to 4 days or frozen for up to 1 month.)

Beef Oxtail Soup with White Beans, Tomatoes, and Aleppo Pepper (Instant Pot)

PREP TIME: 10 MINUTES / COOK TIME: 1 HOUR / SERVES 6 TO 8

Ingredients

4 pounds oxtails, trimmed
1 teaspoon table salt
1 tablespoon extra-virgin olive oil
1 onion, chopped fine
2 carrots, peeled and chopped fine
¼ cup ground dried Aleppo pepper
6 garlic cloves, minced
2 tablespoons tomato paste
¾ teaspoon dried oregano
½ teaspoon ground cinnamon
½ teaspoon ground cumin
6 cups water
1 (28-ounce) can diced tomatoes, drained
1 (15-ounce) can navy beans, rinsed
1 tablespoon sherry vinegar
¼ cup chopped fresh parsley
½ preserved lemon, pulp and white pith removed, rind rinsed and minced (2 tablespoons)

Directions

Preparing the Ingredients

1.   Pat oxtails dry with paper towels and sprinkle with salt. Using highest sauté function, heat oil in Instant Pot for 5 minutes (or until just smoking). Brown half of oxtails, 4 to 6 minutes per side; transfer to plate. Set aside remaining uncooked oxtails.
2.   Add onion and carrots to fat left in pot and cook, using highest sauté function, until softened, about 5 minutes. Stir in Aleppo pepper, garlic, tomato paste, oregano, cinnamon, and cumin and cook until fragrant, about 30 seconds. Stir in water, scraping up any browned bits, then stir in tomatoes. Nestle remaining uncooked oxtails into pot along with browned oxtails and add any accumulated juices.
3.   Lock lid in place and close pressure release valve. Select high pressure cook function and cook for 45 minutes. Turn off Instant Pot and quick-release pressure. Carefully remove lid, allowing steam to escape away from you.
4.   Transfer oxtails to cutting board, let cool slightly, then shred into bite-size pieces using 2 forks; discard bones and excess fat. Strain broth through fine-mesh strainer into large container; return solids to now-empty pot. Using wide, shallow spoon, skim excess fat from surface of liquid; return to pot.
5.   Stir shredded oxtails and any accumulated juices and beans into pot. Using highest sauté function, cook until soup is heated through, about 5 minutes. Stir in vinegar and parsley and season with salt and pepper to taste. Serve, passing preserved lemon separately.

Chopped Greek Antipasto Salad

PREP TIME: 20 MINUTES / COOK TIME: NONE / SERVES 6

Ingredients

1 head Bibb lettuce or ½ head romaine lettuce, chopped (about 2½ cups)
¼ cup loosely packed chopped basil leaves
1 (15-ounce) can chickpeas, drained and rinsed
1 (14-ounce) can artichoke hearts, drained and halved
1 pint grape tomatoes, halved (about 1½ cups)
1 seedless cucumber, peeled and chopped (about 1½ cups)
½ cup cubed feta cheese (about 2 ounces)
1 (2.25-ounce) can sliced black olives (about ½ cup)
For the dressing
3 tablespoons extra-virgin olive oil
1 tablespoon red wine vinegar
1 tablespoon freshly squeezed lemon juice (from about ½ small lemon)
1 tablespoon chopped fresh oregano or ½ teaspoon dried oregano
1 teaspoon honey
¼ teaspoon freshly ground black pepper

Directions

Preparing the Ingredients

1.   In a medium bowl, toss the lettuce and basil together. Spread out on a large serving platter or in a large salad bowl. Arrange the chickpeas, artichoke hearts, tomatoes, cucumber, feta, and olives in piles next to each other on top of the lettuce layer.
2.   In a small pitcher or bowl, whisk together the oil, vinegar, lemon juice, oregano, honey, and pepper. Serve on the side with the salad, or drizzle over all the ingredients right before serving.
3.   Take this dressing to the next level and make a quick oregano oil infusion. Put the oil and oregano in a small skillet over medium-low heat. Let it cook for 5 minutes, stirring occasionally. Remove from the heat and strain through a fine mesh strainer.

Roasted Golden Beet, Avocado, and Watercress Salad

PREP TIME: 15 MINUTES / COOK TIME: 1 HOUR/ SERVES 4

Ingredients

1 bunch (about 1½ pounds) golden beets
1 tablespoon extra-virgin olive oil
1 tablespoon white wine vinegar
½ teaspoon kosher salt
¼ teaspoon freshly ground black pepper
1 bunch (about 4 ounces) watercress
1 avocado, peeled, pitted, and diced
¼ cup crumbled feta cheese
¼ cup walnuts, toasted
1 tablespoon fresh chives, chopped

Directions

Preparing the Ingredients

1.   Preheat the oven to 425°F. Wash and trim the beets (cut an inch above the beet root, leaving the long tail if desired), then wrap each beet individually in foil. Place the beets on a baking sheet and roast until fully cooked, 45 to 60 minutes depending on the size of each beet. Start checking at 45 minutes; if easily pierced with a fork, the beets are cooked.

2.   Remove the beets from the oven and allow them to cool. Under cold running water, slough off the skin. Cut the beets into bite-size cubes or wedges.
3.   In a large bowl, whisk together the olive oil, vinegar, salt, and black pepper. Add the watercress and beets and toss well. Add the avocado, feta, walnuts, and chives and mix gently.

Mediterranean Potato Salad

PREP TIME: 10 MINUTES / COOK TIME: 20 MINUTES/ SERVES 6

Ingredients
2 pounds Yukon Gold baby potatoes, cut into 1-inch cubes
3 tablespoons freshly squeezed lemon juice (from about 1 medium lemon)
3 tablespoons extra-virgin olive oil
1 tablespoon olive brine
¼ teaspoon kosher or sea salt
1 (2.25-ounce) can sliced olives (about ½ cup)
1 cup sliced celery (about 2 stalks) or fennel
2 tablespoons chopped fresh oregano
2 tablespoons torn fresh mint

Directions
Preparing the Ingredients
1.   In a medium saucepan, cover the potatoes with cold water until the waterline is one inch above the potatoes. Set over high heat, bring the potatoes to a boil, then turn down the heat to medium-low. Simmer for 12 to 15 minutes, until the potatoes are just fork tender.
While the potatoes are cooking, in a small bowl, whisk together the lemon juice, oil, olive brine, and salt.
2.   Drain the potatoes in a colander and transfer to a serving bowl. Immediately pour about 3 tablespoons of the dressing over the potatoes. Gently mix in the olives and celery.
3.   Before serving, gently mix in the oregano, mint, and the remaining dressing.

Wild Rice Salad with Chickpeas and Pickled Radish

PREP TIME: 20 MINUTES / COOK TIME: 45 MINUTES/ SERVES 4

Ingredients
1 cup water
4 ounces (⅔ cup) wild rice
¼ teaspoon kosher salt
1 bunch radishes (6 to 8 small), sliced thin
½ cup white wine vinegar
½ teaspoon kosher salt
2 tablespoons extra-virgin olive oil
2 tablespoons white wine vinegar
½ teaspoon pure maple syrup
½ teaspoon kosher salt
¼ teaspoon freshly ground black pepper
1 (15-ounce) can no-salt-added or low-sodium chickpeas, rinsed and drained
1 bulb fennel, diced

¼ cup walnuts, chopped and toasted
¼ cup crumbled feta cheese
¼ cup currants
2 tablespoons fresh dill, chopped

Directions
Preparing the Ingredients
1.   Bring the water, rice, and salt to a boil in a medium saucepan. Cover, reduce the heat, and simmer for 45 minutes.
2.   In a medium bowl, combine the radishes, vinegar, and salt. Let sit for 15 to 30 minutes.
In a large bowl, whisk together the olive oil, vinegar, maple syrup, salt, and black pepper.
While still warm, add the rice to the bowl with the dressing and mix well.
3.   Add the chickpeas, fennel, walnuts, feta, currants, and dill. Mix well.
Garnish with the pickled radishes before serving.

Chop Chop Salad

PREP TIME: 15 MINUTES / COOK TIME: NONE/ SERVES 6

Ingredients
2 heads romaine lettuce, chopped
3 cups chopped skinless cooked chicken breast
1 cup canned or jarred (in water) artichoke hearts, drained, rinsed, and chopped
2 tomatoes, chopped
2 zucchini, chopped
½ red onion, finely chopped
3 ounces mozzarella cheese, chopped
⅓ cup unsweetened nonfat plain Greek yogurt
1 tablespoon Dijon mustard
2 tablespoons extra-virgin olive oil
Zest of 1 lemon
3 garlic cloves, minced
2 tablespoons chopped fresh basil leaves
2 tablespoons chopped fresh chives
½ teaspoon sea salt
⅛ teaspoon freshly ground black pepper

Directions
Preparing the Ingredients
1.   In a large bowl, combine the lettuce, chicken, artichoke hearts, tomatoes, zucchini, red onion, and mozzarella.
2.   In a small bowl, whisk the yogurt, mustard, olive oil, lemon zest, garlic, basil, chives, sea salt, and pepper.
Toss the dressing with the salad before serving.

Fig and Arugula Salad

PREP TIME: 15 MINUTES / COOK TIME: 30 MINUTES / SERVES 2

Ingredients
3 cups arugula
4 fresh, ripe figs (or 4 to 6 dried figs), stemmed and sliced
2 tablespoons olive oil
3 very thin slices prosciutto, trimmed of any fat and sliced lengthwise into 1-inch strips

¼ cup pecan halves, lightly toasted
2 tablespoons crumbled blue cheese
1 to 2 tablespoons balsamic glaze
Directions
Preparing the Ingredients
1. In a large bowl, toss the arugula and figs with the olive oil.
2. Place the prosciutto on a microwave-safe plate and heat it on high in the microwave for 60 seconds, or until it just starts to crisp.
Add the crisped prosciutto, pecans, and blue cheese to the bowl. Toss the salad lightly.
3. Drizzle with the balsamic glaze.

Quinoa with Zucchini, Mint, and Pistachios
PREP TIME: 20 TO 30 MINUTES / COOK TIME: 20 MINUTES/ SERVES 4
Ingredients
1½ cups water
1 cup quinoa
¼ teaspoon kosher salt
2 tablespoons extra-virgin olive oil
1 zucchini, thinly sliced into rounds
6 small radishes, sliced
1 shallot, julienned
¾ teaspoon kosher salt
¼ teaspoon freshly ground black pepper
2 garlic cloves, sliced
Zest of 1 lemon
2 tablespoons lemon juice
¼ cup fresh mint, chopped
¼ cup fresh basil, chopped
¼ cup pistachios, shelled and toasted
Directions
 Preparing the Ingredients. Bring the water, quinoa, and salt to a boil in a medium saucepan. Reduce to a simmer, cover, and cook for 10 to 12 minutes. Fluff with a fork. Heat the olive oil in a large skillet or sauté pan over medium-high heat. Add the zucchini, radishes, shallot, salt, and black pepper, and sauté for 7 to 8 minutes. Add the garlic and cook 30 seconds to 1 minute more. In a large bowl, combine the lemon zest and lemon juice. Add the quinoa and mix well. Add the cooked zucchini mixture and mix well. Add the mint, basil, and pistachios and gently mix.

Panzanella
PREP TIME: 15 MINUTES / COOK TIME: 8 MINUTES/ SERVES 4
Ingredients
6 tablespoons extra-virgin olive oil, divided
4 whole-grain bread slices, crusts removed, cut into pieces
1 cup yellow cherry tomatoes, halved
1 cup red cherry tomatoes, halved
1 plum tomato, cut into wedges
½ red onion, very thinly sliced
¼ cup chopped fresh basil leaves
1 tablespoon capers, drained and rinsed
¼ cup red wine vinegar

2 garlic cloves, minced
½ teaspoon Dijon mustard
½ teaspoon sea salt
¼ teaspoon freshly ground black pepper
Directions
Preparing the Ingredients. In a large skillet over medium-high heat, heat 2 tablespoons of olive oil until it shimmers.
Add the bread and cook for 6 to 8 minutes, stirring occasionally, until crisp and browned. Drain and cool the bread on paper towels. In a large bowl, combine the cooled bread, yellow, red, and plum tomatoes, red onion, basil, and capers. In a small bowl, whisk the remaining 4 tablespoons of olive oil with the vinegar, garlic, mustard, sea salt, and pepper. Toss with the salad and serve.

Summer Panzanella Salad
PREP TIME: 15 MINUTES / COOK TIME: 10 MINUTES, PLUS 15 MINUTES TO REST/ SERVES 2
Ingredients
1 ear corn on the cob, peeled and shucked
4 slices stale French baguette
½ pint cherry or grape tomatoes, halved
1 medium sweet pepper, seeded and cut into 1-inch pieces
1 medium avocado, pitted and cut into cubes
4 very thin slices of sweet onion, cut crosswise into thin rings
½ cup fresh whole basil leaves
2 ounces mini mozzarella balls (ciliegine), halved or quartered
¼ cup honey balsamic dressing
Cooking spray
Directions
Preparing the Ingredients
1. Heat the grill to medium-high heat (about 350°F) and lightly spray the cooking grates with cooking spray.
2. Grill the corn for 10 minutes, or until it is lightly charred all around. Grill the bread for 30 to 45 seconds on each side, or until it has grill marks. Let the corn sit until it's cool enough to handle. Cut the kernels off the cob and place them in a large bowl. Cut the bread into chunks and add it to the bowl.
3. Add the tomatoes, sweet pepper, avocado, onion, basil, mozzarella, and dressing to the bowl, and toss lightly to combine. Let the salad sit for about 15 minutes in the refrigerator, so the bread can soften and the flavors can blend.
This is best served shortly after it's prepared.

Sicilian Fish Stew(Instant Pot)
PREP TIME: 23 MINUTES / COOK TIME: 22 MINUTES/ SERVES 4 TO 6
Ingredients
2 tablespoons extra-virgin olive oil
2 onions, chopped fine
1 teaspoon table salt
½ teaspoon pepper

1 teaspoon minced fresh thyme or ¼ teaspoon dried
Pinch red pepper flakes
4 garlic cloves, minced, divided
1 (28-ounce) can whole peeled tomatoes, drained with juice reserved, chopped coarse
1 (8-ounce) bottle clam juice
¼ cup dry white wine
¼ cup golden raisins
2 tablespoons capers, rinsed
1½ pounds skinless swordfish steak, 1 to 1½ inches thick, cut into 1-inch pieces
¼ cup pine nuts, toasted
¼ cup minced fresh mint
1 teaspoon grated orange zest

Directions

1.   Using highest sauté function, heat oil in Instant Pot until shimmering. Add onions, salt, and pepper and cook until onions are softened, about 5 minutes. Stir in thyme, pepper flakes, and three-quarters of garlic and cook until fragrant, about 30 seconds. Stir in tomatoes and reserved juice, clam juice, wine, raisins, and capers. Nestle swordfish into pot and spoon some cooking liquid over top.
2.   Lock lid in place and close pressure release valve. Select high pressure cook function and cook for 1 minute. Turn off Instant Pot and quick-release pressure. Carefully remove lid, allowing steam to escape away from you.
3.   Combine pine nuts, mint, orange zest, and remaining garlic in bowl. Season stew with salt and pepper to taste. Sprinkle individual portions with pine nut mixture before serving.

Pastina Chicken soup with kale

PREP TIME: 5 MINUTES / COOK TIME: 25 MINUTES/ MAKES 3 CUPS / SERVES 6

Ingredients

1 tablespoon extra-virgin olive oil
2 garlic cloves, minced (about 1 teaspoon)
3 cups packed chopped kale (center ribs removed)
1 cup minced carrots (about 2 carrots)
8 cups low-sodium or no-salt-added chicken (or vegetable) broth
¼ teaspoon kosher or sea salt
¼ teaspoon freshly ground black pepper
¾ cup (6 ounces) uncooked acini de pepe or pastina pasta
2 cups shredded cooked chicken (about 12 ounces)
3 tablespoons grated Parmesan cheese

Directions

1.   **Preparing the Ingredients.** In a large stockpot over medium heat, heat the oil. Add the garlic and cook for 30 seconds, stirring frequently. Add the kale and carrots and cook for 5 minutes, stirring occasionally.
2.   Add the broth, salt, and pepper, and turn the heat to high. Bring the broth to a boil, and add the pasta. Lower the heat to medium and cook for 10 minutes, or until the pasta is cooked through, stirring every few minutes so the pasta doesn't stick to the

bottom. Add the chicken, and cook for 2 more minutes to warm through.
Ladle the soup into six bowls, top each with ½ tablespoon of cheese, and serve.

Italian White Bean Salad with Bell Peppers

PREP TIME: 15 MINUTES / COOK TIME: 20 MINUTES / SERVES 4

Ingredients

2 tablespoons extra-virgin olive oil
2 tablespoons white wine vinegar
½ shallot, minced
½ teaspoon kosher salt
¼ teaspoon freshly ground black pepper
3 cups cooked cannellini beans, or 2 (15-ounce) cans no-salt-added or low-sodium cannellini beans, drained and rinsed
2 celery stalks, diced
½ red bell pepper, diced
¼ cup fresh parsley, chopped
¼ cup fresh mint, chopped

Directions

Preparing the Ingredients

1.   In a large bowl, whisk together the olive oil, vinegar, shallot, salt, and black pepper.
2.   Add the beans, celery, red bell pepper, parsley, and mint; mix well.
To make this salad a heartier lunch or dinner, mix in a cooked whole grain such as farro or sorghum.

Simple Summer Gazpacho

PREP TIME: 15 MINUTES (PLUS 1 HOUR TO CHILL) / COOK TIME: NONE/ SERVES 4

Ingredients

6 tomatoes, chopped
3 garlic cloves, minced
2 red bell peppers, finely chopped
1 red onion, finely chopped
3 cups tomato juice
¼ cup red wine vinegar
¼ cup extra-virgin olive oil
¼ cup basil leaves, torn
½ teaspoon sea salt
¼ teaspoon freshly ground black pepper

Directions

1.   In a blender or food processor, combine the tomatoes, garlic, red bell peppers, red onion, tomato juice, vinegar, olive oil, basil, sea salt, and pepper. Pulse for 20 to 30 (1-second) pulses until blended. Chill for 1 hour before serving.
2.   Spice it up by adding 1 chile pepper or a few dashes of your favorite hot sauce.

Watermelon Feta Salad

PREP TIME: 10 MINUTES / COOK TIME: NONE/ MAKES 3 CUPS / SERVES 2

Ingredients

3 cups packed arugula
2½ cups watermelon, cut into bite-size cubes

2 ounces feta cheese, crumbled
2 tablespoons balsamic glaze
Directions
Preparing the Ingredients
1.   Divide the arugula between two plates. Divide the watermelon cubes between the beds of arugula. Sprinkle 1 ounce of the feta over each salad.
2.   Drizzle about 1 tablespoon of the glaze (or more if desired) over each salad.

Roasted Red Pepper Soup with Smoked Paprika and Cilantro Yogurt

PREP TIME: 15 MINUTES / COOK TIME: 10 MINUTES/ SERVES 6
Ingredients
½ cup whole-milk yogurt
3 tablespoons minced fresh cilantro
1 teaspoon lime juice
Salt and pepper
8 red bell peppers, cored and flattened
1 tablespoon extra-virgin olive oil
2 garlic cloves, minced
1 red onion, chopped
½ teaspoon ground cumin
½ teaspoon smoked paprika
2 tablespoons tomato paste
1 tablespoon all-purpose flour
4 cups chicken or vegetable broth, plus extra as needed
1 bay leaf
½ cup half-and-half
2 tablespoons dry sherry
Directions
Preparing the Ingredients
1.   Whisk yogurt, 1 tablespoon cilantro, and lime juice together in bowl. Season with salt and pepper to taste. Cover and refrigerate until needed.
2.   Adjust oven rack 3 inches from broiler element and heat broiler. Spread half of peppers skin side up on aluminum foil–lined baking sheet. Broil until skin is charred and puffed but flesh is still firm, 8 to 10 minutes, rotating sheet halfway through broiling. Transfer broiled peppers to bowl, cover with plastic wrap or foil, and let steam until skins peel off easily, 10 to 15 minutes. Repeat with remaining peppers. Peel broiled peppers, discarding skins, and chop coarse.
3.   Cook oil and garlic together in Dutch oven over low heat, stirring constantly, until garlic is foamy, sticky, and straw-colored, 6 to 8 minutes. Stir in onion and ¼ teaspoon salt, increase heat to medium, and cook until softened, about 5 minutes.
4.   Stir in cumin and paprika and cook until fragrant, about 30 seconds. Stir in tomato paste and flour and cook for 1 minute. Slowly whisk in broth, scraping up any browned bits and smoothing out any lumps. Stir in bay leaf and chopped peppers, bring to simmer, and cook until peppers are very tender, 5 to 7 minutes.

5.   Discard bay leaf. Working in batches, process soup in blender until smooth, about 2 minutes. Return soup to clean pot and stir in half-and-half and sherry. Heat soup gently over low heat until hot (do not boil) and adjust consistency with extra hot broth as needed. Stir in remaining 2 tablespoons cilantro and season with salt and pepper to taste. Serve, drizzling individual portions with yogurt mixture.

Mushroom Barley Soup

PREP TIME: 5 MINUTES / COOK TIME: 25 MINUTES/ MAKES 6 CUPS / SERVES 6
Ingredients
2 tablespoons extra-virgin olive oil
1 cup chopped onion (about ½ medium onion)
1 cup chopped carrots (about 2 carrots)
5½ cups chopped mushrooms (about 12 ounces)
6 cups low-sodium or no-salt-added vegetable broth
1 cup uncooked pearled barley
¼ cup red wine
2 tablespoons tomato paste
4 sprigs fresh thyme or ½ teaspoon dried thyme
1 dried bay leaf
6 tablespoons grated Parmesan cheese
Directions
Preparing the Ingredients
1.   In a large stockpot over medium heat, heat the oil. Add the onion and carrots and cook for 5 minutes, stirring frequently. Turn up the heat to medium-high and add the mushrooms. Cook for 3 minutes, stirring frequently.
2.   Add the broth, barley, wine, tomato paste, thyme, and bay leaf. Stir, cover the pot, and bring the soup to a boil. Once it's boiling, stir a few times, reduce the heat to medium-low, cover, and cook for another 12 to 15 minutes, until the barley is cooked through.
Remove the bay leaf and serve in soup bowls with 1 tablespoon of cheese sprinkled on top of each.

French Lentil Salad with Parsley and Mint

PREP TIME: 20 MINUTES / COOK TIME: 25 MINUTES / SERVES 4
Ingredients
1 cup French lentils
1 garlic clove, smashed
1 dried bay leaf
2 tablespoons extra-virgin olive oil
2 tablespoons red wine vinegar
½ teaspoon ground cumin
½ teaspoon kosher salt
¼ teaspoon freshly ground black pepper
2 celery stalks, diced small
1 bell pepper, diced small
½ red onion, diced small
¼ cup fresh parsley, chopped
¼ cup fresh mint, chopped
Directions
Preparing the Ingredients

1. Put the lentils, garlic, and bay leaf in a large saucepan. Cover with water by about 3 inches and bring to a boil. Reduce the heat, cover, and simmer until tender, 20 to 30 minutes.
2. Drain the lentils to remove any remaining water after cooking. Remove the garlic and bay leaf.
3. In a large bowl, whisk together the olive oil, vinegar, cumin, salt, and black pepper. Add the celery, bell pepper, onion, parsley, and mint and toss to combine. Add the lentils and mix well.

Butternut Squash Soup

PREP TIME: 15 MINUTES / COOK TIME: 35 MINUTES/ MAKES 4 CUPS / SERVES 4
Ingredients
2 tablespoons extra-virgin olive oil
1 onion, chopped
1 carrot, chopped
1 celery stalk, chopped
4 cups unsalted vegetable broth
3 cups chopped butternut squash
1 teaspoon dried thyme
½ teaspoon sea salt
¼ teaspoon freshly ground black pepper
Directions
Preparing the Ingredients
1. In a large pot over medium-high heat, heat the olive oil until it shimmers. Add the onion, carrot, and celery. Cook for 5 to 7 minutes, stirring occasionally, until the vegetables begin to brown. Add the broth, squash, thyme, sea salt, and pepper. Bring to a simmer and reduce the heat to medium. Simmer for 20 to 30 minutes until the squash is soft.
2. Purée the soup using an immersion blender, food processor, or blender.

Easy Pasta Fagioli Soup

PREP TIME: 5 MINUTES / COOK TIME: 25 MINUTES/ SERVES 6
Ingredients
2 tablespoons extra-virgin olive oil
½ cup chopped onion (about ¼ onion)
3 garlic cloves, minced (about 1½ teaspoons)
1 tablespoon minced fresh rosemary or 1 teaspoon dried rosemary
¼ teaspoon crushed red pepper
4 cups low-sodium or no-salt-added vegetable broth
2 (15.5-ounce) cans cannellini, great northern, or light kidney beans, undrained
1 (28-ounce) can low-sodium or no-salt-added crushed tomatoes
2 tablespoons tomato paste
8 ounces uncooked short pasta, such as ditalini, tubetti, or elbows
6 tablespoons grated Parmesan cheese (about 1½ ounces)
Directions
1. In a large stockpot over medium heat, heat the oil. Add the onion and cook for 4 minutes, stirring frequently. Add the garlic, rosemary, and crushed red pepper. Cook for 1 minute, stirring frequently. Add the broth, canned beans with their liquid, tomatoes, and tomato paste. Simmer for 5 minutes.
2. To thicken the soup, carefully transfer 2 cups to a blender. Purée, then stir it back into the pot.
3. Bring the soup to a boil over high heat. Mix in the pasta, and lower the heat to a simmer. Cook the pasta for the amount of time recommended on the box, stirring every few minutes to prevent the pasta from sticking to the pot. Taste the pasta to make sure it is cooked through (it could take a few more minutes than the recommended cooking time, since it's cooking with other ingredients).
4. Ladle the soup into bowls, top each with 1 tablespoon of grated cheese, and serve.

Roasted Cauliflower and Arugula Salad with Pomegranate and Pine Nuts

PREP TIME: 5 MINUTES / COOK TIME: 20 MINUTES/ SERVES 4
Ingredients
1 head cauliflower, trimmed and cut into 1-inch florets
2 tablespoons extra-virgin olive oil, plus more for drizzling (optional)
1 teaspoon ground cumin
½ teaspoon kosher salt
¼ teaspoon freshly ground black pepper
5 ounces arugula
⅓ cup pomegranate seeds
¼ cup pine nuts, toasted
Directions
1. **Preparing the Ingredients**
Preheat the oven to 425°F. Line a baking sheet with parchment paper or foil. In a large bowl, combine the cauliflower, olive oil, cumin, salt, and black pepper.
2. **Cooking**
Spread in a single layer on the prepared baking sheet and roast for 20 minutes, tossing halfway through. Divide the arugula among 4 plates. Top with the cauliflower, pomegranate seeds, and pine nuts. Serve with Lemon Vinaigrette dressing or a simple drizzle of olive oil.

White Bean Soup with Kale

PREP TIME: 5 MINUTES / COOK TIME: 20 MINUTES/ SERVES 6
Ingredients
2 tablespoons extra-virgin olive oil
8 ounces Italian chicken sausage (uncooked), sliced
1 onion, chopped 1 carrot, chopped
1 red bell pepper, seeded and chopped
3 garlic cloves, minced
6 cups unsalted vegetable broth
1 (14-ounce) can white beans, drained
4 cups chopped kale
1 teaspoon dried thyme
½ teaspoon sea salt
¼ teaspoon freshly ground black pepper
Pinch red pepper flakes

Directions
Preparing the Ingredients
1. In a large pot over medium-high heat, heat the olive oil until it shimmers.
2. Add the sausage and cook for about 5 minutes, stirring occasionally, until browned. Remove the sausage from the pot with a slotted spoon and set it aside.
Add the onion, carrot, and red bell pepper to the oil remaining in the pot. Cook for about 5 minutes, stirring occasionally, until the vegetables are soft. Add the garlic and cook for 30 seconds, stirring constantly.
3. Stir in the broth, beans, kale, thyme, sea salt, pepper, and red pepper flakes. Bring to a simmer. Reduce the heat to low and simmer for about 5 minutes more until the kale is soft.
Return the sausage to the pot. Cook for 1 minute more until the sausage heats through. Serve immediately.

Citrus Fennel Salad

PREP TIME: 15 MINUTES / COOK TIME: 0 MINUTES/ SERVES 2
Ingredients
2 tablespoons fresh orange juice
3 tablespoons olive oil
1 tablespoon blood orange vinegar, other orange vinegar, or cider vinegar
1 tablespoon honey
Salt
Freshly ground black pepper
For the salad
2 cups packed baby kale
1 medium navel or blood orange, segmented
½ small fennel bulb, stems and leaves removed, sliced into matchsticks
3 tablespoons toasted pecans, chopped
2 ounces goat cheese, crumbled
Directions
1. **Preparing the Ingredients**
Divide the baby kale, orange segments, fennel, pecans, and goat cheese evenly between two plates. Drizzle half of the dressing over each salad. Baby kale is usually sold prewashed in bags. If it's only available mixed with other greens, That works fine. Combine the orange juice, olive oil, vinegar, and honey in a small bowl and whisk to combine. Season with salt and pepper. Set the dressing aside.

Roasted Carrot Soup with Parmesan Croutons

PREP TIME: 10 MINUTES / COOK TIME: 20 MINUTES/ SERVES 4
Ingredients
2 pounds carrots, unpeeled, cut into ½-inch slices (about 6 cups)
2 tablespoons extra-virgin olive oil, divided
1 cup chopped onion (about ½ medium onion)
2 cups low-sodium or no-salt-added vegetable (or chicken) broth
2½ cups water
1 teaspoon dried thyme
¼ teaspoon crushed red pepper
¼ teaspoon kosher or sea salt
4 thin slices whole-grain bread
⅓ cup freshly grated Parmesan cheese (about 1 ounce)
Directions
1. **Preparing the Ingredients**
Place one oven rack about four inches below the broiler element. Place two large, rimmed baking sheets in the oven on any oven rack. Preheat the oven to 450°F.
2. **Cooking**
In a large bowl, toss the carrots with 1 tablespoon of oil to coat. With oven mitts, carefully remove the baking sheets from the oven and evenly distribute the carrots on both sheets. Bake for 20 minutes, until the carrots are just fork tender, stirring once halfway through. The carrots will still be somewhat firm. Remove the carrots from the oven, and turn the oven to the high broil setting. While the carrots are roasting, in a large stockpot over medium-high heat, heat 1 tablespoon of oil. Add the onion and cook for 5 minutes, stirring occasionally. Add the broth, water, thyme, crushed red pepper, and salt. Bring to a boil, cover, then remove the pan from the heat until the carrots have finished roasting.
Add the roasted carrots to the pot, and blend with an immersion blender (or use a regular blender—carefully pour in the hot soup in batches, then return the soup to the pot). Heat the soup for about 1 minute over medium-high heat, until warmed through. Turn the oven to the high broil setting. Place the bread on the baking sheet. Sprinkle the cheese evenly across the slices of bread. Broil the bread 4 inches below the heating element for 1 to 2 minutes, or until the cheese melts, watching carefully to prevent burning. Cut the bread into bite-size croutons. Divide the soup evenly among four bowls, top each with the Parmesan croutons, and serve.

Red Gazpacho

PREP TIME: 15 MINUTES / COOK TIME: 0 MINUTES/ SERVES 4
Ingredients
2 pounds tomatoes, cut into chunks
1 bell pepper, cut into chunks
1 cucumber, cut into chunks
1 small red onion, cut into chunks
1 garlic clove, smashed
2 teaspoons sherry vinegar
½ teaspoon kosher salt
¼ teaspoon freshly ground black pepper
⅓ cup extra-virgin olive oil
Lemon juice (optional)
¼ cup fresh chives, chopped, for garnish
Directions

Preparing the Ingredients

In a high-speed blender or Vitamix, add the tomatoes, bell pepper, cucumber, onion, garlic, vinegar, salt, and black pepper. Blend until smooth. With the motor running, add the olive oil and purée until smooth. Add more vinegar or a spritz of lemon juice if needed. Garnish with the chives. Any herbs will go nicely with this refreshing cold soup. Use parsley, basil, or whatever you like in place of the chives.

Lentil Soup

PREP TIME: 10 MINUTES / COOK TIME: 20 MINUTES/ SERVES 4

Ingredients

2 tablespoons extra-virgin olive oil
2 onions, chopped
2 celery stalks, chopped
2 carrots, chopped
4 garlic cloves, minced
1 (14-ounce) can lentils, drained
2 bay leaves
6 cups unsalted vegetable broth
1 teaspoon sea salt
¼ teaspoon freshly ground black pepper
Pinch red pepper flakes
¼ cup red wine vinegar

Directions
Preparing the Ingredients

1.　　In a large pot over medium-high heat, heat the olive oil until it shimmers.
2.　　Add the onions, celery, and carrots. Cook for 5 to 10 minutes, stirring occasionally, until the vegetables are soft.
Add the garlic and cook for 30 seconds, stirring constantly.
3.　　Stir in the lentils, bay leaves, broth, sea salt, pepper, and red pepper flakes. Bring to a simmer. Reduce the heat to medium-low and simmer for 10 minutes, stirring occasionally.
Remove and discard the bay leaves. Stir in the vinegar and serve.

Avgolemono (Lemon Chicken Soup)

PREP TIME: 15 MINUTES / COOK TIME: 60 MINUTES/ SERVES 2 WITH 2 SERVINGS FOR LEFTOVERS

Ingredients

½ large onion
2 medium carrots
1 celery stalk
1 garlic clove
5 cups low-sodium chicken stock
¼ cup brown rice
1½ cups (about 5 ounces) shredded rotisserie chicken
3 tablespoons freshly squeezed lemon juice
1 egg yolk
2 tablespoons chopped fresh dill
2 tablespoons chopped fresh parsley
Salt

Directions
Preparing the Ingredients

1.　　Place the onion, carrots, celery, and garlic in a food processor fitted with the chopping blade and pulse it until the vegetables are minced. You can also mince them by hand.
Add the vegetables and chicken stock to a stockpot or Dutch oven and bring it to a boil over high heat.
2.　　Reduce the heat to medium-low and add the rice, shredded chicken and lemon juice. Cover, and let the soup simmer for 40 minutes, or until the rice is cooked.
3.　　In a small bowl, whisk the egg yolk lightly. Very slowly, while whisking with one hand, pour about ½ of a ladle of the broth into the egg yolk to warm, or temper, the yolk. Slowly add another ladle of broth and continue to whisk.
Remove the soup from the heat and pour the whisked egg yolk–broth mixture into the pot. Stir well to combine.
Add the fresh dill and parsley. Season with salt, and serve.

Paella Soup

PREP TIME: 5 MINUTES / COOK TIME: 25 MINUTES/ SERVES 6

Ingredients

1 cup frozen green peas
2 tablespoons extra-virgin olive oil
1 cup chopped onion (about ½ medium onion)
1½ cups coarsely chopped red bell pepper (about 1 large pepper)
1½ cups coarsely chopped green bell pepper (about 1 large pepper)
2 garlic cloves, chopped (about 1 teaspoon)
1 teaspoon ground turmeric
1 teaspoon dried thyme
2 teaspoons smoked paprika
2½ cups uncooked instant brown rice
2 cups low-sodium or no-salt-added chicken broth
2½ cups water
1 (28-ounce) can low-sodium or no-salt-added crushed tomatoes
1 pound fresh raw medium shrimp (or frozen raw shrimp completely thawed), shells and tails removed

Directions
Preparing the Ingredients

1.　　Put the frozen peas on the counter to partially thaw as the soup is being prepared.
2.　　In a large stockpot over medium-high heat, heat the oil. Add the onion, red and green bell peppers, and garlic. Cook for 8 minutes, stirring occasionally. Add the turmeric, thyme, and smoked paprika, and cook for 2 minutes more, stirring often. Stir in the rice, broth, and water. Bring to a boil over high heat. Cover, reduce the heat to medium-low, and cook for 10 minutes.
3.　　Stir the peas, tomatoes, and shrimp into the soup. Cook for 4 to 6 minutes, until the shrimp is cooked, turning from gray to pink and white. The

soup will be very thick, almost like stew, when ready to serve.

Roasted Eggplant Soup

PREP TIME: 15 MINUTES / COOK TIME: 40 MINUTES/ SERVES 6

Ingredients

2 pounds (1 to 2 medium to large) eggplant, halved lengthwise
2 beefsteak tomatoes, halved
2 onions, halved
4 garlic cloves, smashed
4 rosemary sprigs
2 tablespoons extra-virgin olive oil
1 to 2 cups no-salt-added vegetable stock
1 teaspoon pure maple syrup
1 teaspoon ground cumin
1 teaspoon ground coriander
1 teaspoon kosher salt
¼ teaspoon freshly ground black pepper
Lemon juice (optional)

Directions

Preparing the Ingredients

1. Preheat the oven to 400°F. Line two baking sheets with parchment paper or foil. Lightly spray with olive oil cooking spray. Spread the eggplant, tomatoes, onions, and garlic on the prepared baking sheets, cut-side down. Nestle the rosemary sprigs among the vegetables. Drizzle with the olive oil and roast for 40 minutes, checking halfway through and removing the garlic before it gets brown.
2. When cool enough to touch, remove the eggplant flesh and tomato flesh from the skin and add to a high-powered blender, food processor, or Vitamix.
3. Add the rosemary leaves, onions, garlic, 1 cup of the vegetable stock, maple syrup, cumin, coriander, salt, and black pepper. Purée until smooth.
4. The soup should be thick and creamy. If the soup is too thick, add another cup of stock slowly, until your desired consistency is reached. Spritz with lemon juice, if desired.

Chicken and Vegetable Soup

PREP TIME: 10 MINUTES / COOK TIME: 20 MINUTES/ SERVES 8

Ingredients

2 tablespoons extra-virgin olive oil
12 ounces boneless, skinless chicken breast, sliced
2 carrots, chopped
1 onion, chopped
1 red bell pepper, seeded and chopped
1 fennel bulb, chopped
5 garlic cloves, minced
6 cups unsalted chicken broth
1 (14-ounce) can crushed tomatoes, undrained
2 zucchini, chopped
1 tablespoon dried Italian seasoning
½ teaspoon sea salt
¼ teaspoon freshly ground black pepper

Directions

Preparing the Ingredients

1. In a large pot over medium-high heat, heat the olive oil until it shimmers.
2. Add the chicken and cook for about 5 minutes, stirring occasionally, until browned. Remove the chicken from the pot with a slotted spoon and set it aside.
Add the carrots, onion, red bell pepper, and fennel to the oil remaining in the pot. Cook for about 5 minutes, stirring occasionally, until the vegetables are soft.
Add the garlic and cook for 30 seconds, stirring constantly.
Stir in the broth, tomatoes, zucchini, Italian seasoning, sea salt, and pepper.
Bring to a boil, stirring occasionally. Reduce the heat and simmer for about 5 minutes more until the vegetables are soft.
Return the chicken to the pot. Cook for 1 minute more until the chicken heats through. Serve immediately.
To prepare the fennel bulb, cut off the stalks and reserve them for another use.
Cut the core from the bottom of the fennel in a "V" shape and discard. Halve the fennel lengthwise and chop. The remaining stalks can be added to salads, or cooked down like an onion to add to any dish.

Lentil Sweet Potato Soup

PREP TIME: 5 MINUTES / COOK TIME: 30 MINUTES/ SERVES 6

Ingredients

1 tablespoon extra-virgin olive oil
1 onion, diced
1 carrot, diced
1 celery stalk, diced
1 sweet potato, unpeeled and diced
1 cup green or brown lentils
1 dried bay leaf
1 teaspoon ground turmeric
1 teaspoon ground cumin
1 teaspoon kosher salt
¼ teaspoon freshly ground black pepper
4 cups no-salt-added vegetable stock

Directions

Preparing the Ingredients

Heat the olive oil in a large stockpot over medium-high heat. Add the onion, carrot, celery, and sweet potato and sauté 5 to 6 minutes. Add the lentils, bay leaf, turmeric, cumin, salt, and black pepper and cook for 30 seconds to 1 minute more.
Add the stock, bring to a boil, then lower the heat to low, and simmer, covered for 20 to 30 minutes, or until the lentils and sweet potato are tender.If you find the soup becoming thick and stew-like, feel free to add additional stock or water as it cooks. Herbs are a welcome addition to most dishes. If you have any fresh herbs, feel free to mix in ¼ cup chopped to the finished soup.

Zucchini and Meatball Soup

PREP TIME: 20 MINUTES / COOK TIME: 25 MINUTES/ SERVES 6

Ingredients

12 ounces ground turkey
1 yellow onion, grated and squeezed of excess water
1 tablespoon dried Italian seasoning
1 teaspoon garlic powder
1 teaspoon sea salt, divided
½ teaspoon freshly ground black pepper, divided
2 tablespoons extra-virgin olive oil
1 red onion, chopped
5 garlic cloves, minced
6 cups unsalted chicken broth
1 (14-ounce) can chopped tomatoes, drained
3 medium zucchini, chopped or spiralized
¼ cup chopped fresh basil leaves

Directions

Preparing the Ingredients

1.   In a medium bowl, mix together the turkey, yellow onion, Italian seasoning, garlic powder, ½ teaspoon of sea salt, and ¼ teaspoon of pepper. On a plate, form the mixture into ¾-inch balls and set aside.
In a large pot over medium-high heat, heat the olive oil until it shimmers.
2.   Add the red onion and cook for about 5 minutes, stirring occasionally, until soft.
Add the garlic and cook for 30 seconds, stirring constantly.
Stir in the broth, tomatoes, remaining ½ teaspoon of salt, and remaining ¼ teaspoon of pepper. Bring to a boil. Add the meatballs and return to a boil. Reduce the heat to medium-low. Simmer for about 15 minutes, stirring occasionally, until the meatballs are cooked through.
Add the zucchini and cook for about 3 minutes more, until soft.
Stir in the basil just before serving.

Turmeric Red Lentil Soup

PREP TIME: 5 MINUTES / COOK TIME: 30 MINUTES/ SERVES 6

Ingredients

1 tablespoon extra-virgin olive oil
1 teaspoon ground cumin
1 teaspoon ground coriander
1 teaspoon ground turmeric
1 teaspoon kosher salt
¼ teaspoon freshly ground black pepper
1 tablespoon no-salt-added tomato paste
1 onion, diced
1 carrot, diced
1 celery stalk, diced
3 garlic cloves, minced
4 cups no-salt-added vegetable stock
2 cups water
1 cup red lentils
3 tablespoons lemon juice
¼ cup fresh parsley, chopped

Directions

Preparing the Ingredients

1.   Heat the olive oil in a large stock pot over medium-high heat. Add the cumin, coriander, turmeric, salt, and black pepper and cook, stirring, for 30 seconds. Add the tomato paste and cook, stirring, for 30 seconds to 1 minute. Add the onion, carrot, and celery and sauté 5 to 6 minutes. Add the garlic and sauté 30 seconds.
2.   Add the vegetable stock, water, and lentils and bring to a boil. Turn down the heat to low, and simmer, covering partially, until the lentils are tender, about 20 minutes. Mix in the lemon juice and parsley.

Tuscan Bean Soup with Kale

PREP TIME: 5 MINUTES / COOK TIME: 25 MINUTES/ SERVES 4

Ingredients

2 tablespoons extra-virgin olive oil
1 onion, diced
1 carrot, diced
1 celery stalk, diced
1 teaspoon kosher salt
4 cups no-salt-added vegetable stock
1 (15-ounce) can no-salt-added or low-sodium cannellini beans, drained and rinsed
1 tablespoon fresh thyme, chopped
1 tablespoon fresh sage, chopped
1 tablespoon fresh oregano, chopped
¼ teaspoon freshly ground black pepper
1 bunch kale, stemmed and chopped
¼ cup grated Parmesan cheese (optional)

Directions

Preparing the Ingredients

1.   Heat the olive oil in a large pot over medium-high heat. Add the onion, carrot, celery, and salt and sauté until translucent and slightly golden, 5 to 6 minutes. Add the vegetable stock, beans, thyme, sage, oregano, and black pepper and bring to a boil. Turn down the heat to low, and simmer for 10 minutes. Stir in the kale and let it wilt, about 5 minutes. Sprinkle 1 tablespoon Parmesan cheese over each bowl before serving, if desired.

All-Purpose Chicken Broth (Instant Pot)

PREP TIME: 60 MINUTES / COOK TIME: 60 MINUTES/ SERVES 6 TO 8

Ingredients

3 pounds chicken wings
1 tablespoon vegetable oil
1 onion, chopped
3 garlic cloves, lightly crushed and peeled
12 cups water, divided
½ teaspoon table salt
3 bay leaves

Directions

1.   Pat chicken wings dry with paper towels. Using highest sauté function, heat oil in Instant Pot for 5 minutes (or until just smoking). Brown half of chicken wings on all sides, about 10 minutes;

transfer to bowl. Repeat with remaining chicken wings; transfer to bowl. Add onion to fat left in pot and cook until softened and well browned, 8 to 10 minutes. Stir in garlic and cook until fragrant, about 30 seconds. Stir in 1 cup water, scraping up any browned bits. Stir in remaining 11 cups water, salt, bay leaves, and chicken and any accumulated juices.

2.	Lock lid in place and close pressure release valve. Select high pressure cook function and cook for 1 hour. Turn off Instant Pot and let pressure release naturally for 15 minutes. Quick-release any remaining pressure, then carefully remove lid, allowing steam to escape away from you.

3.	Strain broth through fine-mesh strainer into large container, pressing on solids to extract as much liquid as possible; discard solids. Using wide, shallow spoon, skim excess fat from surface of broth. (Broth can be refrigerated for up to 4 days or frozen for up to 2 months.)

Moroccan-Style Chickpea Soup

PREP TIME: 5 MINUTES / COOK TIME: 30 MINUTES/ SERVES 4 TO 6

Ingredients

3 tablespoons extra-virgin olive oil
1 onion, chopped fine
1 teaspoon sugar
Salt and pepper
4 garlic cloves, minced
½ teaspoon hot paprika
¼ teaspoon saffron threads, crumbled
¼ teaspoon ground ginger
¼ teaspoon ground cumin
2 (15-ounce) cans chickpeas, rinsed
1 pound red potatoes, unpeeled, cut into ½-inch pieces
1 (14.5-ounce) can diced tomatoes
1 zucchini, cut into ½-inch pieces
3½ cups chicken or vegetable broth
¼ cup minced fresh parsley or mint
Lemon wedges

Directions

Preparing the Ingredients

1.	Heat oil in Dutch oven over medium-high heat until shimmering. Add onion, sugar, and ½ teaspoon salt and cook until onion is softened, about 5 minutes. Stir in garlic, paprika, saffron, ginger, and cumin and cook until fragrant, about 30 seconds. Stir in chickpeas, potatoes, tomatoes and their juice, zucchini, and broth. Bring to simmer and cook, stirring occasionally, until potatoes are tender, 20 to 30 minutes.

2.	Using wooden spoon, mash some of potatoes against side of pot to thicken soup. Off heat, stir in parsley and season with salt and pepper to taste. Serve with lemon wedges.

VEGETARIAN MAINS

Socca Pan Pizza with Herbed Ricotta, Fresh Tomato, and Balsamic Glaze

PREP TIME: 15 MINUTES / COOK TIME: 15 MINUTES/ SERVES 2

Ingredients
1 cup chickpea flour
1 teaspoon baking powder
½ teaspoon salt
½ teaspoon garlic powder
½ teaspoon onion powder
1½ teaspoons Italian seasoning herb mix, divided
2 tablespoons grated Parmesan cheese
Up to 1 cup warm water
Olive oil, enough to coat the bottom of a skillet
½ cup ricotta cheese
1 ripe tomato, thinly sliced
Balsamic glaze

Directions
1.   Preparing the Ingredients
Preheat the oven to 425°F and set the rack to the middle position.

While the oven is heating, combine the chickpea flour, baking powder, salt, garlic powder, onion powder, 1 teaspoon of the Italian seasoning herb mix, and the Parmesan cheese in a medium bowl.

Add most of the water and whisk to combine. The batter should be a pourable consistency like pancake batter, but not as thin as a crepe batter. You may not need all of the water.

2.   Cooking.
Heat a large (10- to 12-inch) nonstick or cast iron skillet on the stovetop over medium-high heat and add the oil.

When the pan is hot, pour the batter into the pan and let it cook for a minute, until bubbles start to form. Transfer the pan to the oven and let it cook for 10 minutes, or until the batter starts to turn golden around the edges and looks set.

In a small bowl, combine the ricotta cheese and the remaining ½ teaspoon of Italian seasoning herb mix. Remove the pan from the oven and gently spread the ricotta over the crust. Top with the sliced tomatoes and return to the oven for another 2 minutes to let the cheese melt.

Use a spatula to remove the dough from the pan. Drizzle it with balsamic glaze, slice, and serve.

Beet and Watercress Salad with Orange and Dill (Instant Pot)

PREP TIME: 5 MINUTES / COOK TIME: 8 MINUTES / SERVES 4

Ingredients
2 pounds beets, scrubbed, trimmed, and cut into ¾-inch pieces
½ cup water
1 teaspoon caraway seeds
½ teaspoon table salt
1 cup plain Greek yogurt
1 small garlic clove, minced to paste
5 ounces (5 cups) watercress, torn into bite-size pieces
1 tablespoon extra-virgin olive oil, divided, plus extra for drizzling
1 tablespoon white wine vinegar, divided
1 teaspoon grated orange zest plus 2 tablespoons juice
¼ cup hazelnuts, toasted, skinned, and chopped
¼ cup coarsely chopped fresh dill
Coarse sea salt

Directions
Preparing the Ingredients
1.   Combine beets, water, caraway seeds, and table salt in Instant Pot. Lock lid in place and close pressure release valve. Select high pressure cook function and cook for 8 minutes. Turn off Instant Pot and quick-release pressure. Carefully remove lid, allowing steam to escape away from you.

2.   Using slotted spoon, transfer beets to plate; set aside to cool slightly. Combine yogurt, garlic, and 3 tablespoons beet cooking liquid in bowl; discard remaining cooking liquid. In large bowl toss watercress with 2 teaspoons oil and 1 teaspoon vinegar. Season with table salt and pepper to taste.

3.   Spread yogurt mixture over surface of serving dish. Arrange watercress on top of yogurt mixture, leaving 1-inch border of yogurt mixture. Add beets to now-empty large bowl and toss with orange zest and juice, remaining 2 teaspoons vinegar, and remaining 1 teaspoon oil. Season with table salt and pepper to taste. Arrange beets on top of watercress mixture. Drizzle with extra oil and sprinkle with hazelnuts, dill, and sea salt.

Cauliflower Steaks with Olive Citrus Sauce

PREP TIME: 15 MINUTES / COOK TIME: 30 MINUTES / SERVES 4

Ingredients
1 or 2 large heads cauliflower (at least 2 pounds, enough for 4 portions)
⅓ cup extra-virgin olive oil
¼ teaspoon kosher salt
⅛ teaspoon ground black pepper
Juice of 1 orange
Zest of 1 orange
¼ cup black olives, pitted and chopped
1 tablespoon Dijon or grainy mustard
1 tablespoon red wine vinegar
½ teaspoon ground coriander

Directions
1.   Preparing the Ingredients
Preheat the oven to 400°F. Line a baking sheet with parchment paper or foil.

Cut off the stem of the cauliflower so it will sit upright. Slice it vertically into four thick slabs. Place

the cauliflower on the prepared baking sheet. Drizzle with the olive oil, salt, and black pepper.
2.   **Cooking**. Bake for about 30 minutes, turning over once, until tender and golden brown. In a medium bowl, combine the orange juice, orange zest, olives, mustard, vinegar, and coriander; mix well. Serve the cauliflower warm or at room temperature with the sauce.

Easy Brussels Sprouts Hash

PREP TIME: 5 MINUTES / COOK TIME: 20 MINUTES/ SERVES 4
Ingredients
3 tablespoons extra-virgin olive oil
1 onion, finely chopped
1 pound Brussels sprouts, bottoms trimmed off.
½ teaspoon caraway seeds
½ teaspoon sea salt
⅛ teaspoon freshly ground black pepper
¼ cup red wine vinegar
1 tablespoon Dijon mustard
1 tablespoon honey
3 garlic cloves, minced
Directions
Preparing the Ingredients
1.   In a large skillet over medium-high heat, heat the olive oil until it shimmers.
Add the onion, Brussels sprouts, caraway seeds, sea salt, and pepper. Cook for 7 to 10 minutes, stirring occasionally, until the Brussels sprouts begin to brown.
2.   While the Brussels sprouts cook, whisk the vinegar, mustard, and honey in a small bowl and set aside.
Add the garlic to the skillet and cook for 30 seconds, stirring constantly.
Add the vinegar mixture to the skillet. Cook for about 5 minutes, stirring, until the liquid reduces by half. An easy way to prepare the sprouts is to carefully grate them on a box grater, or use a mandoline set at ¼ inch with a guard. It allows you to have pieces of similar size so they cook evenly.

Caprese-Stuffed Portobellos

PREP TIME: 10 MINUTES / COOK TIME: 20 MINUTES/ SERVES 2
Ingredients
1 tablespoon olive oil, plus extra for drizzling
½ pint cherry or grape tomatoes
¼ teaspoon salt
Pinch freshly ground black pepper
3 medium garlic cloves, minced
4 to 5 large fresh basil leaves, thinly sliced, divided
2 large portobello mushrooms, stems removed
4 pieces mini mozzarella balls (ciliegine), halved
1 tablespoon grated Parmesan cheese
Directions
1.   **Preparing the Ingredients**. Preheat the oven to 350°F.

2.   **Cooking**. Heat 1 tablespoon of the olive oil in a sauté pan over medium-high heat. Add the tomatoes, salt, and pepper. Pierce a few of the tomatoes as they cook so they give off some juice. Cover and let the tomatoes soften for about 10 minutes. When the tomatoes are mostly softened and begin to break down, add the minced garlic and most of the basil—reserve about 2 teaspoons of basil to garnish at the end. Cook for 30 seconds and then remove from the heat.
Oil a baking pan and place the mushrooms gill-side up. If desired, season with salt and pepper. Divide the tomato mixture and the mozzarella balls between the mushrooms. Sprinkle the grated Parmesan cheese evenly over each and, if desired, drizzle the mushrooms with olive oil. Bake them for 20 minutes, or until the mushrooms are softened. If desired, place them under the broiler to brown the cheese a bit. Garnish with the remaining fresh basil.

Meze Plate with Hummus, Spiced Carrots, and Arugula(Instant Pot)

PREP TIME: 20 MINUTES / COOK TIME: 20 MINUTES/ MAKES ¼ CUP / SERVES 4
Ingredients
2 pounds carrots, peeled
½ cup chicken or vegetable broth
3 tablespoons Harissa (this page), divided
½ teaspoon table salt
2 ounces (2 cups) baby arugula
1 tablespoon extra-virgin olive oil
2 teaspoons lemon juice
1½ cups Hummus (this page)
½ cup Quick Pickled Onions (this page)
2 tablespoons roasted pepitas
Directions
Preparing the Ingredients
1.   Cut carrots into 3-inch lengths. Leave thin pieces whole and halve larger pieces lengthwise. Combine carrots, broth, 1 tablespoon Harissa, and salt in Instant Pot. Lock lid in place and close pressure release valve. Select high pressure cook function and cook for 1 minute. Turn off Instant Pot and quick-release pressure. Carefully remove lid, allowing steam to escape away from you; drain carrots.
2.   Gently toss arugula with oil and lemon juice in bowl. Season with salt and pepper to taste. Spread portion of Hummus over bottom of individual serving plates. Using slotted spoon, arrange carrots on top and drizzle with remaining 2 tablespoons Harissa. Top with arugula, pickled onions, and pepitas.

Walnut Pesto Zoodles

PREP TIME: 15 MINUTES / COOK TIME: 10 MINUTES/ MAKES ¼ CUP / SERVES 4
Ingredients
4 medium zucchini (makes about 8 cups of zoodles)
¼ cup extra-virgin olive oil, divided

2 garlic cloves, minced (about 1 teaspoon), divided
½ teaspoon crushed red pepper
¼ teaspoon freshly ground black pepper, divided
¼ teaspoon kosher or sea salt, divided
2 tablespoons grated Parmesan cheese, divided
1 cup packed fresh basil leaves
¾ cup walnut pieces, divided

Directions

1.   Preparing the Ingredients
Make the zucchini noodles (zoodles) using a spiralizer or your vegetable peeler to make ribbons (run the peeler down the zucchini to make long strips). In a large bowl, gently mix to combine the zoodles with 2 tablespoon of oil, 1 minced garlic clove, all the crushed red pepper, ⅛ teaspoon of black pepper, and ⅛ teaspoon of salt. Set aside.

2.   Cooking
In a large skillet over medium-high heat, heat ½ tablespoon of oil. Add half of the zoodles to the pan and cook for 5 minutes, stirring every minute or so. Pour the cooked zoodles into a large serving bowl, and repeat with another ½ tablespoon of oil and the remaining zoodles. Add those zoodles to the serving bowl when they are done cooking. While the zoodles are cooking, make the pesto. If you're using a food processor, add the remaining minced garlic clove, ⅛ teaspoon of black pepper, and ⅛ teaspoon of salt, 1 tablespoon of Parmesan, all the basil leaves, and ¼ cup of walnuts. Turn on the processor, and slowly drizzle the remaining 2 tablespoons of oil into the opening until the pesto is completely blended. If you're using a high-powered blender, add the 2 tablespoons of oil first and then the rest of the pesto ingredients. Pulse until the pesto is completely blended. Add the pesto to the zoodles along with the remaining 1 tablespoon of Parmesan and the remaining ½ cup of walnuts. Mix together well and serve.

Pistachio Mint Pesto Pasta

PREP TIME: 10 MINUTES / COOK TIME: 10 MINUTES/ MAKES ¼ CUP / SERVES 4

Ingredients
8 ounces whole-wheat pasta
1 cup fresh mint
½ cup fresh basil
⅓ cup unsalted pistachios, shelled
1 garlic clove, peeled
½ teaspoon kosher salt
Juice of ½ lime
⅓ cup extra-virgin olive oil

Directions

Preparing the Ingredients
1.   Cook the pasta according to the package directions. Drain, reserving ½ cup of the pasta water, and set aside.
2.   In a food processor, add the mint, basil, pistachios, garlic, salt, and lime juice. Process until the pistachios are coarsely ground. Add the olive oil

in a slow, steady stream and process until incorporated.
3.   In a large bowl, mix the pasta with the pistachio pesto; toss well to incorporate. If a thinner, more saucy consistency is desired, add some of the reserved pasta water and toss well.

Roasted Asparagus with Lemon and Pine Nuts
PREP TIME: 5 MINUTES / COOK TIME: 20 MINUTES/ SERVES 4

Ingredients
1pound asparagus, trimmed
2 tablespoons extra-virgin olive oil
Juice of 1 lemon
Zest of 1 lemon
¼ cup pine nuts
½ teaspoon sea salt
⅛ teaspoon freshly ground black pepper

Directions

1.   Preparing the Ingredients
Preheat the oven to 425°F.
In a large bowl, toss the asparagus with the olive oil, lemon juice and zest, pine nuts, sea salt, and pepper. Spread in a roasting pan in an even layer.

2.   Cooking
Roast for about 20 minutes until the asparagus is browned.

Mushroom-Leek Tortilla de Patatas

PREP TIME: 30 MINUTES / COOK TIME:30 MINUTES, PLUS 5 MINUTES TO REST/ SERVES 2

Ingredients
1 tablespoon olive oil
1 cup thinly sliced leeks (from 1 leek, light green part only)
4 ounces baby bella (cremini) mushrooms, stemmed and sliced (about 1 cup)
1 small potato, peeled, sliced ¼-inch thick
5 large eggs, beaten
½ cup milk
1 teaspoon Dijon mustard
½ teaspoon dried thyme
½ teaspoon salt
Pinch freshly ground black pepper
3 ounces Gruyère cheese, shredded

Directions

Preparing the Ingredients
1.   Preheat the oven to 350°F and set the rack to the middle position.
Heat the olive oil in a large sauté pan (nonstick is best) over medium-high heat. Add the leeks, mushrooms, and potato slices and sauté until the leeks are golden and the potatoes start to brown, about 10 minutes.
2.   Reduce the heat to medium-low, cover the pan, and let the vegetables cook for another 10 minutes, or until the potatoes begin to soften. If the potato slices stick to the bottom of the pan, add 1 to 2 tablespoons of water to the pan, but be careful because it may splatter.

3. While the vegetables are cooking, combine the beaten eggs, milk, mustard, thyme, salt, pepper, and cheese in a medium bowl and whisk everything together.

4. When the potatoes are soft enough to pierce with a fork or knife, turn off the heat. Transfer the cooked vegetables to an oiled 8-inch oven-safe pan (nonstick is best) and arrange them in a nice layer along the bottom and slightly up the sides of the pan. Alternatively, you can use a glass pie or quiche dish. A smaller pan will give you a nice, tall, moist omelet.

5. Pour the egg mixture over the vegetables and give it a light shake or tap to distribute the eggs evenly through the vegetables.

Bake the tortilla for 25 to 30 minutes, or until the eggs are set and the top is golden and puffed. Remove it from the oven, and let it sit for 5 minutes before cutting into it.

Rustic Garlic Toasts with Stewed Tomatoes, Shaved Fennel, and Burrata (Instnt Pot)

PREP TIME: 5 MINUTES / COOK TIME: 8 MINUTES/ SERVES 4

Ingredients
2 tablespoons extra-virgin olive oil, divided, plus extra for drizzling
5 garlic cloves, sliced thin
1½ teaspoons fennel seeds, lightly cracked
1 (28-ounce) can whole peeled tomatoes, drained with juice reserved, halved
⅛ teaspoon table salt
8 ounces burrata cheese, room temperature
1 fennel bulb, stalks discarded, bulb halved, cored, and sliced thin
4 ounces (4 cups) baby arugula
1 recipe Garlic Toasts (this page)
Balsamic glaze
Coarse sea salt

Directions
Preparing the Ingredients
1. Using highest sauté function, cook 1 tablespoon oil, garlic, and fennel seeds in Instant Pot until fragrant and garlic is light-golden brown, about 3 minutes. Stir in tomatoes and reserved juice and table salt. Lock lid in place and close pressure release valve. Select high pressure cook function and cook for 2 minutes.

2. Turn off Instant Pot and quick-release pressure. Carefully remove lid, allowing steam to escape away from you. Continue to cook tomato mixture using highest sauté function until sauce is slightly thickened, about 5 minutes.

3. Place burrata on plate and cut into rough 1½-inch pieces, collecting creamy liquid. Toss fennel and arugula with remaining 1 tablespoon oil in large bowl. Season with table salt and pepper to taste. Arrange toasts on individual serving plates and top with tomato mixture, fennel-arugula salad, and

burrata and any accumulated liquid. Drizzle with glaze and extra oil, and sprinkle with sea salt.

Cauliflower Steaks with Eggplant Relish

PREP TIME: 5 MINUTES / COOK TIME: 25 MINUTES / SERVES 4

Ingredients
2 small heads cauliflower (about 3 pounds)
¼ teaspoon kosher or sea salt
¼ teaspoon smoked paprika
Extra-virgin olive oil, divided

Directions
1. **Preparing the Ingredients**
Place a large, rimmed baking sheet in the oven. Preheat the oven to 400°F with the pan inside. Stand one head of cauliflower on a cutting board, stem-end down. With a long chef's knife, slice down through the very center of the head, including the stem. Starting at the cut edge, measure about 1 inch and cut one thick slice from each cauliflower half, including as much of the stem as possible, to make two cauliflower "steaks." Reserve the remaining cauliflower for another use. Repeat with the second cauliflower head.

Dry each steak well with a clean towel. Sprinkle the salt and smoked paprika evenly over both sides of each cauliflower steak.

2. **Cooking**
In a large skillet over medium-high heat, heat 2 tablespoons of oil. When the oil is very hot, add two cauliflower steaks to the pan and cook for about 3 minutes, until golden and crispy. Flip and cook for 2 more minutes. Transfer the steaks to a plate. Use a pair of tongs to hold a paper towel and wipe out the pan to remove most of the hot oil (which will contain a few burnt bits of cauliflower). Repeat the cooking process with the remaining 2 tablespoons of oil and the remaining two steaks.

Using oven mitts, carefully remove the baking sheet from the oven and place the cauliflower on the baking sheet. Roast in the oven for 12 to 15 minutes, until the cauliflower steaks are just fork tender; they will still be somewhat firm. Serve the steaks with the Eggplant Relish Spread, baba ghanoush, or the homemade ketchup from our Italian Baked Beans recipe.

Burst Cherry Tomato Sauce with Angel Hair Pasta

PREP TIME: 10 MINUTES / COOK TIME: 20 MINUTES/ SERVES 4

Ingredients
8 ounces angel hair pasta
2 tablespoons extra-virgin olive oil
3 garlic cloves, minced
3 pints cherry tomatoes
½ teaspoon kosher salt
¼ teaspoon red pepper flakes
¾ cup fresh basil, chopped
1 tablespoon white balsamic vinegar (optional)

¼ cup grated Parmesan cheese (optional)
Directions
1.   Cook the pasta according to the package directions. Drain and set aside.
2.   Heat the olive oil in a skillet or large sauté pan over medium-high heat. Add the garlic and sauté for 30 seconds. Add the tomatoes, salt, and red pepper flakes and cook, stirring occasionally, until the tomatoes burst, about 15 minutes.
3.   Remove from the heat and add the pasta and basil. Toss together well. (For out-of-season tomatoes, add the vinegar, if desired, and mix well.) Serve with the grated Parmesan cheese, if desired.

Citrus Sautéed Spinach

PREP TIME: 5 MINUTES / COOK TIME: 5 MINUTES/ SERVES 4
Ingredients
2 tablespoons extra-virgin olive oil
4 cups fresh baby spinach
1 teaspoon orange zest
¼ cup freshly squeezed orange juice
½ teaspoon sea salt
⅛ teaspoon freshly ground black pepper
Directions
1.   **Preparing the Ingredients**
In a large skillet over medium-high heat, heat the olive oil until it shimmers. Add the spinach and orange zest. Cook for about 3 minutes, stirring occasionally, until the spinach wilts. Stir in the orange juice, sea salt, and pepper. Cook for 2 minutes more, stirring occasionally. Serve hot. Before serving, add ¼ cup chopped walnuts for crunch. The recipe also works with kale or Swiss chard, but increase the cooking time to about 10 minutes.

Gnocchi with Creamy Butternut Squash and Blue Cheese Sauce

PREP TIME: 10 MINUTES / COOK TIME: 20 MINUTES/ SERVES 2
Ingredients
5 ounces frozen diced butternut squash
¼ cup low-sodium vegetable stock
Pinch salt
Pinch nutmeg
Pinch cayenne pepper
Pinch freshly ground black pepper
8 ounces prepared, packaged gnocchi
1 tablespoon olive oil
1 garlic clove, minced
2 fresh sage leaves
1 ounce Gorgonzola Dolce or other mild blue cheese
1 tablespoon heavy cream (optional)
Directions
1.   **Preparing the Ingredients**
In a saucepan, bring the butternut squash and vegetable stock to a boil. Cover, and reduce the heat to medium-low. Simmer for 10 minutes, or until the squash is very tender.

Transfer the squash and vegetable stock to a blender. Add the salt, nutmeg, cayenne, and black pepper, and blend on low speed until it's completely smooth. (Make sure your blender is no more than half full or the hot liquid may erupt through the lid.) Taste and add additional salt if needed. Set the squash aside. Using the same saucepan, cook the gnocchi according to package directions. While the gnocchi cooks, heat the olive oil in a large sauté pan over medium-high heat. Add the garlic and sage and sauté for 45 seconds, just until the garlic and sage are fragrant. Carefully add the puréed squash to the sauté pan. Stir in the cheese and cream, if using. Add the cooked gnocchi to the pan and gently stir to coat with the sauce. Taste and add any salt, pepper, or another pinch of nutmeg as needed. Remove the sage leaves before serving. Gnocchi are made from potato and flour and they cook very quickly. Make sure you remove them from the heat as soon as the gnocchi float to the top of the pan. I like to use a slotted spoon and scoop them right from the water and into the sauce.

Mediterranean Lentil Sloppy Joes

PREP TIME: 5 MINUTES / COOK TIME: 15 MINUTES/ SERVES 4
Ingredients
1 tablespoon extra-virgin olive oil
1 cup chopped onion (about ½ medium onion)
1 cup chopped bell pepper, any color (about 1 medium bell pepper)
2 garlic cloves, minced (about 1 teaspoon)
1 (15-ounce) can lentils, drained and rinsed
1 (14.5-ounce) can low-sodium or no-salt-added diced tomatoes, undrained
1 teaspoon ground cumin
1 teaspoon dried thyme
¼ teaspoon kosher or sea salt
4 whole-wheat pita breads, split open
1½ cups chopped seedless cucumber (1 medium cucumber)
1 cup chopped romaine lettuce
Directions
Preparing the Ingredients
1.   In a medium saucepan over medium-high heat, heat the oil. Add the onion and bell pepper and cook for 4 minutes, stirring frequently. Add the garlic and cook for 1 minute, stirring frequently. Add the lentils, tomatoes (with their liquid), cumin, thyme, and salt. Turn the heat to medium and cook, stirring occasionally, for 10 minutes, or until most of the liquid has evaporated.
2.   Stuff the lentil mixture inside each pita. Lay the cucumbers and lettuce on top of the lentil mixture and serve.

Baked Tofu with Sun-Dried Tomatoes and Artichokes

PREP TIME: 15 MINUTES, PLUS 15 MINUTES TO MARINATE / COOK TIME: 30 MINUTES/ SERVES 4

Ingredients

1 (16-ounce) package extra-firm tofu, drained and patted dry, cut into 1-inch cubes
2 tablespoons extra-virgin olive oil, divided
2 tablespoons lemon juice, divided
1 tablespoon low-sodium soy sauce or gluten-free tamari
1 onion, diced
½ teaspoon kosher salt
2 garlic cloves, minced
1 (14-ounce) can artichoke hearts, drained
8 sun-dried tomato halves packed in oil, drained and chopped
¼ teaspoon freshly ground black pepper
1 tablespoon white wine vinegar
Zest of 1 lemon
¼ cup fresh parsley, chopped

Directions

1. **Preparing the Ingredients.** Preheat the oven to 400°F. Line a baking sheet with foil or parchment paper.
In a bowl, combine the tofu, 1 tablespoon of the olive oil, 1 tablespoon of the lemon juice, and the soy sauce. Allow to sit and marinate for 15 to 30 minutes.
2. **Cooking.** Arrange the tofu in a single layer on the prepared baking sheet and bake for 20 minutes, turning once, until light golden brown. Heat the remaining 1 tablespoon olive oil in a large skillet or sauté pan over medium heat. Add the onion and salt; sauté until translucent, 5 to 6 minutes. Add the garlic and sauté for 30 seconds. Add the artichoke hearts, sun-dried tomatoes, and black pepper and sauté for 5 minutes.
Add the white wine vinegar and the remaining 1 tablespoon lemon juice and deglaze the pan, scraping up any brown bits. Remove the pan from the heat and stir in the lemon zest and parsley. Gently mix in the baked tofu.

Mashed Cauliflower

PREP TIME: 10 MINUTES / COOK TIME: 15 MINUTES / SERVES 4

Ingredients

4 cups cauliflower florets
¼ cup skim milk
¼ cup (2 ounces) grated Parmesan cheese
2 tablespoons butter
2 tablespoons extra-virgin olive oil
½ teaspoon sea salt
⅛ teaspoon freshly ground black pepper

Directions

1. **Preparing the Ingredients.** In a large pot over medium-high, cover the cauliflower with water and bring it to a boil. Reduce the heat to medium-low, cover, and simmer for about 10 minutes until the cauliflower is soft.
Drain the cauliflower and return it to the pot. Add the milk, cheese, butter, olive oil, sea salt, and pepper. Using a potato masher, mash until smooth.

Roasted Ratatouille Pasta

PREP TIME: 10 MINUTES / COOK TIME: 20 MINUTES/ SERVES 2

Ingredients

1 small eggplant (about 8 ounces)
1 small zucchini
1 portobello mushroom
1 Roma tomato, halved
½ medium sweet red pepper, seeded
½ teaspoon salt, plus additional for the pasta water
1 teaspoon Italian herb seasoning
1 tablespoon olive oil
2 cups farfalle pasta (about 8 ounces)
2 tablespoons minced sun-dried tomatoes in olive oil with herbs
2 tablespoons prepared pesto

Directions

1. **Preparing the Ingredients**
Slice the ends off the eggplant and zucchini. Cut them lengthwise into ½-inch slices.
Place the eggplant, zucchini, mushroom, tomato, and red pepper in a large bowl and sprinkle with ½ teaspoon of salt. Using your hands, toss the vegetables well so that they're covered evenly with the salt. Let them rest for about 10 minutes.
While the vegetables are resting, preheat the oven to 400°F and set the rack to the bottom position. Line a baking sheet with parchment paper. When the oven is hot, drain off any liquid from the vegetables and pat them dry with a paper towel. Add the Italian herb seasoning and olive oil to the vegetables and toss well to coat both sides.
2. **Cooking**.
Lay the vegetables out in a single layer on the baking sheet. Roast them for 15 to 20 minutes, flipping them over after about 10 minutes or once they start to brown on the underside. When the vegetables are charred in spots, remove them from the oven. While the vegetables are roasting, fill a large saucepan with water. Add salt and cook the pasta according to package directions. Drain the pasta, reserving ½ cup of the pasta water.
When cool enough to handle, cut the vegetables into large chunks (about 2 inches) and add them to the hot pasta.
Stir in the sun-dried tomatoes and pesto and toss everything well.

Gorgonzola Sweet Potato Burgers

PREP TIME: 10 MINUTES / COOK TIME: 15 MINUTES/ SERVES 4

Ingredients

1 large sweet potato (about 8 ounces)
2 tablespoons extra-virgin olive oil, divided
1 cup chopped onion (about ½ medium onion)
1 cup old-fashioned rolled oats
1 large egg
1 tablespoon balsamic vinegar
1 tablespoon dried oregano
1 garlic clove

¼ teaspoon kosher or sea salt
½ cup crumbled Gorgonzola or blue cheese (about 2 ounces)
Salad greens or 4 whole-wheat rolls, for serving (optional)

Directions

1.   **Preparing the Ingredients**
Using a fork, pierce the sweet potato all over and microwave on high for 4 to 5 minutes, until tender in the center. Cool slightly, then slice in half.

While the sweet potato is cooking, in a large skillet over medium-high heat, heat 1 tablespoon of oil. Add the onion and cook for 5 minutes, stirring occasionally.

Using a spoon, carefully scoop the sweet potato flesh out of the skin and put the flesh in a food processor. Add the onion, oats, egg, vinegar, oregano, garlic, and salt. Process until smooth. Add the cheese and pulse four times to barely combine. With your hands, form the mixture into four (½-cup-size) burgers. Place the burgers on a plate, and press to flatten each to about ¾-inch thick.

Wipe out the skillet with a paper towel, then heat the remaining 1 tablespoon of oil over medium-high heat until very hot, about 2 minutes. Add the burgers to the hot oil, then turn the heat down to medium. Cook the burgers for 5 minutes, flip with a spatula, then cook an additional 5 minutes. Enjoy as is or serve on salad greens or whole-wheat rolls.

To make your burgers a uniform size, divide the burger mixture into roughly quarter sections, then pack a portion into a ½-cup measuring cup. Pop each burger out of the measuring cup, then flatten and pack it with your hands into a ¾-inch-thick patty.

Baked Mediterranean Tempeh with Tomatoes and Garlic

PREP TIME: 25 MINUTES, PLUS 4 HOURS TO MARINATE / COOK TIME: 35 MINUTES/ SERVES 4

Ingredients
12 ounces tempeh
¼ cup white wine
2 tablespoons extra-virgin olive oil
2 tablespoons lemon juice
Zest of 1 lemon
¼ teaspoon kosher salt
¼ teaspoon freshly ground black pepper
1 tablespoon extra-virgin olive oil
1 onion, diced
3 garlic cloves, minced
1 (14.5-ounce) can no-salt-added crushed tomatoes
1 beefsteak tomato, diced
1 dried bay leaf
1 teaspoon white wine vinegar
1 teaspoon lemon juice
1 teaspoon dried oregano
1 teaspoon dried thyme
¾ teaspoon kosher salt
¼ cup basil, cut into ribbons

Directions

1.   **Preparing the Ingredients**
Place the tempeh in a medium saucepan. Add enough water to cover it by 1 to 2 inches. Bring to a boil over medim-high heat, cover, and lower heat to a simmer. Cook for 10 to 15 minutes. Remove the tempeh, pat dry, cool, and cut into 1-inch cubes.

In a large bowl, combine the white wine, olive oil, lemon juice, lemon zest, salt, and black pepper. Add the tempeh, cover the bowl, and put in the refrigerator for 4 hours, or up to overnight.

Preheat the oven to 375°F. Place the marinated tempeh and the marinade in a baking dish and cook for 15 minutes.

Heat the olive oil in a large skillet over medium heat. Add the onion and sauté until transparent, 3 to 5 minutes.

Add the garlic and sauté for 30 seconds. Add the crushed tomatoes, beefsteak tomato, bay leaf, vinegar, lemon juice, oregano, thyme, and salt. Mix well. Simmer for 15 minutes.

Add the baked tempeh to the tomato mixture and gently mix together. Garnish with the basil.

Broccoli with Ginger and Garlic

PREP TIME: 10 MINUTES / COOK TIME: 11 MINUTES / SERVES 4

Ingredients
2 tablespoons extra-virgin olive oil
2 cups broccoli florets
1 tablespoon grated fresh ginger
½ teaspoon sea salt
⅛ teaspoon freshly ground black pepper
3 garlic cloves, minced

Directions

1.   **Preparing the Ingredients.** In a large skillet over medium-high heat, heat the olive oil until it shimmers.

2.   Add the broccoli, ginger, sea salt, and pepper. Cook for about 10 minutes, stirring occasionally, until the broccoli is soft and starts to brown. Add the garlic and cook for 30 seconds, stirring constantly. Remove from the heat and serve.

Mushroom Ragù with Parmesan Polenta

PREP TIME: 20 MINUTES / COOK TIME: 45 MINUTES / SERVES 2

Ingredients
½ ounce dried porcini mushrooms (optional but recommended)
2 tablespoons olive oil
1 pound baby bella (cremini) mushrooms, quartered
1 large shallot, minced (about ⅓ cup)
1 garlic clove, minced
1 tablespoon flour
2 teaspoons tomato paste
½ cup red wine
1 cup mushroom stock (or reserved liquid from soaking the porcini mushrooms, if using)
½ teaspoon dried thyme
1 fresh rosemary sprig

1½ cups water
½ teaspoon salt
⅓ cup instant polenta
2 tablespoons grated Parmesan cheese
Directions
1.   Preparing the Ingredients
If using the dried porcini mushrooms, soak them in 1 cup of hot water for about 15 minutes to soften them. When they're softened, scoop them out of the water, reserving the soaking liquid. (I strain it through a coffee filter to remove any possible grit.) Mince the porcini mushrooms.
2.   Cooking
Heat the olive oil in a large sauté pan over medium-high heat. Add the mushrooms, shallot, and garlic, and sauté for 10 minutes, or until the vegetables are wilted and starting to caramelize. Add the flour and tomato paste, and cook for another 30 seconds. Add the red wine, mushroom stock or porcini soaking liquid, thyme, and rosemary. Bring the mixture to a boil, stirring constantly until it thickens. Reduce the heat and let it simmer for 10 minutes. While the mushrooms are simmering, bring the water to a boil in a saucepan and add salt. Add the instant polenta and stir quickly while it thickens. Stir in the Parmesan cheese. Taste and add additional salt if needed. Make sure you buy instant polenta, which cooks in seconds. Regular polenta takes about 45 minutes to cook.

Garlicky Kale and Parsnips with Soft-Cooked Eggs and Pickled Onions (Instant Pot)

PREP TIME: 20 MINUTES / COOK TIME: 9 MINUTES/ SERVES 4
Ingredients
12 ounces parsnips, peeled
2 tablespoons extra-virgin olive oil, plus extra for drizzling
4 garlic cloves, minced
2 pounds kale, stemmed and cut into 1-inch pieces
¾ cup chicken or vegetable broth
½ teaspoon table salt
4 large eggs
¼ cup Quick Pickled Onions
½ cup Lemon-Yogurt Sauce
1 teaspoon ground dried Aleppo pepper
Directions
1.   Preparing the Ingredients
Cut parsnips into 2-inch lengths. Leave thin pieces whole, halve medium pieces lengthwise, and quarter thick pieces lengthwise. Using highest sauté function, cook oil and garlic in Instant Pot until fragrant, about 1 minute. Stir in half of kale and cook until slightly wilted, about 1 minute. Add remaining kale and repeat. Stir in broth and salt, then add parsnips. Lock lid in place and close pressure release valve. Select high pressure cook function and cook for 3 minutes.

Turn off Instant Pot and quick-release pressure. Carefully remove lid, allowing steam to escape away from you. Season kale and parsnips with salt and pepper to taste. Transfer to bowl and cover to keep warm. Discard cooking liquid in pot.
Arrange trivet included with Instant Pot in base of now-empty insert and add 1 cup water. Using highest sauté function, bring water to boil. Set eggs on trivet. Lock lid in place and close pressure release valve. Select high pressure cook function and set cook time for 3 minutes. Cook eggs for 2½ minutes (fully set whites with runny yolks) or 3 minutes (fully set whites with fudgy yolks).
Turn off Instant Pot and quick-release pressure. Carefully remove lid, allowing steam to escape away from you. Using tongs, transfer eggs to separate bowl and place under cold running water for 30 seconds. Drain and peel eggs.
Divide kale and parsnips among individual serving bowls. Top with pickled onions, yogurt sauce, and eggs. Sprinkle with Aleppo pepper and drizzle with extra oil. Serve.

Zucchini-Eggplant Gratin

PREP TIME: 10 MINUTES / COOK TIME: 10 MINUTES / SERVES 6
Ingredients
1 large eggplant, finely chopped (about 5 cups)
2 large zucchini, finely chopped (about 3¾ cups)
¼ teaspoon freshly ground black pepper
¼ teaspoon kosher or sea salt
3 tablespoons extra-virgin olive oil, divided
1 tablespoon all-purpose flour
¾ cup 2% milk
⅓ cup plus 2 tablespoons grated Parmesan cheese, divided
1 cup chopped tomato (about 1 large tomato)
1 cup diced or shredded fresh mozzarella (about 4 ounces)
¼ cup fresh basil leaves
Directions
1.   Preparing the Ingredients
Preheat the oven to 425°F. In a large bowl, toss together the eggplant, zucchini, pepper, and salt.
2.   Cooking.
In a large skillet over medium-high heat, heat 1 tablespoon of oil. Add half the veggie mixture to the skillet. Stir a few times, then cover and cook for 5 minutes, stirring occasionally. Pour the cooked veggies into a baking dish. Place the skillet back on the heat, add 1 tablespoon of oil, and repeat with the remaining veggies. Add the veggies to the baking dish. While the vegetables are cooking, heat the milk in the microwave for 1 minute. Set aside.
Place a medium saucepan over medium heat. Add the remaining tablespoon of oil and flour, and whisk together for about 1 minute, until well blended. Slowly pour the warm milk into the oil mixture, whisking the entire time. Continue to whisk frequently until the mixture thickens a bit. Add ⅓

cup of Parmesan cheese, and whisk until melted. Pour the cheese sauce over the vegetables in the baking dish and mix well.

Gently mix in the tomatoes and mozzarella cheese. Roast in the oven for 10 minutes, or until the gratin is almost set and not runny. Garnish with the fresh basil leaves and the remaining 2 tablespoons of Parmesan cheese before serving.

Roasted Portobello Mushrooms with Kale and Red Onion

PREP TIME: 15 MINUTES, PLUS 15 MINUTES TO MARINATE / COOK TIME: 30 MINUTES/ SERVES 4
Ingredients
¼ cup white wine vinegar
3 tablespoons extra-virgin olive oil, divided
½ teaspoon honey
¾ teaspoon kosher salt, divided
¼ teaspoon freshly ground black pepper
4 large (4 to 5 ounces each) portobello mushrooms, stems removed
1 red onion, julienned
2 garlic cloves, minced
1 (8-ounce) bunch kale, stemmed and chopped small
¼ teaspoon red pepper flakes
¼ cup grated Parmesan or Romano cheese
Directions
1.   **Preparing the Ingredients**
Line a baking sheet with parchment paper or foil. In a medium bowl, whisk together the vinegar, 1½ tablespoons of the olive oil, honey, ¼ teaspoon of the salt, and the black pepper. Arrange the mushrooms on the baking sheet and pour the marinade over them. Marinate for 15 to 30 minutes.
2.   **Cooking**
Meanwhile, preheat the oven to 400°F. Bake the mushrooms for 20 minutes, turning over halfway through.
Heat the remaining 1½ tablespoons olive oil in a large skillet or ovenproof sauté pan over medium-high heat. Add the onion and the remaining ½ teaspoon salt and sauté until golden brown, 5 to 6 minutes. Add the garlic and sauté for 30 seconds. Add the kale and red pepper flakes and sauté until the kale cooks down, about 5 minutes.
Remove the mushrooms from the oven and increase the temperature to broil.
Carefully pour the liquid from the baking sheet into the pan with the kale mixture; mix well.
Turn the mushrooms over so that the stem side is facing up. Spoon some of the kale mixture on top of each mushroom. Sprinkle 1 tablespoon Parmesan cheese on top of each.
Broil until golden brown, 3 to 4 minutes.

Balsamic Roasted Carrots

PREP TIME: 10 MINUTES / COOK TIME: 30 MINUTES/ SERVES 4
Ingredients
1½ pounds carrots, quartered lengthwise

2 tablespoons extra-virgin olive oil
¼ teaspoon sea salt
⅛ teaspoon freshly ground black pepper
3 tablespoons balsamic vinegar
Directions
1.   **Preparing the Ingredients**
Preheat the oven to 425°F. In a large bowl, toss the carrots with the olive oil, sea salt, and pepper. Place in a single layer in a roasting pan or on a rimmed baking sheet.
2.   **Cooking.** Roast for 20 to 30 minutes until the carrots are caramelized. Toss with the vinegar and serve.

Braised Fennel with Radicchio, Rear, and Pecorino (Instant Pot)

PREP TIME: 22 MINUTES / COOK TIME: 23 MINUTES/ SERVES 4
Ingredients
6 tablespoons extra-virgin olive oil, divided
2 fennel bulbs (12 ounces each), 2 tablespoons fronds chopped, stalks discarded, bulbs halved, each half cut into 1-inch-thick wedges
¾ teaspoon table salt, divided
½ teaspoon grated lemon zest plus 4 teaspoons juice
5 ounces (5 cups) baby arugula
1 small head radicchio (6 ounces), shredded
1 Bosc or Bartlett pear, quartered, cored, and sliced thin
¼ cup whole almonds, toasted and chopped
Shaved Pecorino Romano cheese
Directions
1.   **Preparing the Ingredients**
Using highest sauté function, heat 2 tablespoons oil in Instant Pot for 5 minutes (or until just smoking). Brown half of fennel, about 3 minutes per side; transfer to plate. Repeat with 1 tablespoon oil and remaining fennel; do not remove from pot.
Return first batch of fennel to pot along with ½ cup water and ½ teaspoon salt. Lock lid in place and close pressure release valve. Select high pressure cook function and cook for 2 minutes. Turn off Instant Pot and quick-release pressure. Carefully remove lid, allowing steam to escape away from you. Using slotted spoon, transfer fennel to plate; discard cooking liquid.
Whisk remaining 3 tablespoons oil, lemon zest and juice, and remaining ¼ teaspoon salt together in large bowl. Add arugula, radicchio, and pear and toss to coat. Transfer arugula mixture to serving dish and arrange fennel wedges on top. Sprinkle with almonds, fennel fronds, and Pecorino.

Grilled Stuffed Portobello Mushrooms

PREP TIME: 5 MINUTES / COOK TIME: 25 MINUTES/ SERVES 6
Ingredients
3 tablespoons extra-virgin olive oil, divided
1 cup diced onion (about ½ medium onion)
2 garlic cloves, minced (about 1 teaspoon)

3 cups chopped mushrooms, any variety
1 large or 2 small zucchini or summer squash, diced (about 2 cups)
1 cup chopped tomato (about 1 large tomato)
1 teaspoon dried oregano
¼ teaspoon crushed red pepper
¼ teaspoon kosher or sea salt
6 large portobello mushrooms, stems and gills removed
Nonstick cooking spray (if needed)
4 ounces fresh mozzarella cheese, shredded

Directions
Preparing the Ingredients
1.   In a large skillet over medium heat, heat 2 tablespoons of oil. Add the onion and cook for 4 minutes, stirring occasionally. Stir in the garlic and cook for 1 minute, stirring often. Stir in the mushrooms, zucchini, tomato, oregano, crushed red pepper, and salt. Cook for 10 minutes, stirring occasionally. Remove from the heat.
2.   While the veggies are cooking, heat the grill or grill pan to medium-high heat.
3.   Brush the remaining tablespoon of oil over the portobello mushroom caps. Place the mushrooms bottom-side (where the stem was removed) down on the grill or pan. Cover and cook for 5 minutes. (If using a grill pan, cover with a sheet of aluminum foil sprayed with nonstick cooking spray.)
4.   Flip the mushroom caps over, and spoon about ½ cup of the cooked vegetable mixture into each cap. Top each with about 2½ tablespoons of mozzarella and additional oregano, if desired.
Cover and grill for 4 to 5 minutes, or until the cheese melts. Remove each portobello with a spatula, and let them sit for about 5 minutes to cool slightly before serving.

Balsamic Marinated Tofu with Basil and Oregano

PREP TIME: 10 MINUTES, PLUS 30 MINUTES TO MARINATE / COOK TIME: 30 MINUTES/ SERVES 4
Ingredients
¼ cup extra-virgin olive oil
¼ cup balsamic vinegar
2 tablespoons low-sodium soy sauce or gluten-free tamari
3 garlic cloves, grated
2 teaspoons pure maple syrup
Zest of 1 lemon
1 teaspoon dried basil
1 teaspoon dried oregano
½ teaspoon dried thyme
½ teaspoon dried sage
¼ teaspoon kosher salt
¼ teaspoon freshly ground black pepper
¼ teaspoon red pepper flakes (optional)
1 (16-ounce) block extra firm tofu, drained and patted dry, cut into ½-inch or 1-inch cubes

Directions
1.   **Preparing the Ingredients**

In a bowl or gallon zip-top bag, mix together the olive oil, vinegar, soy sauce, garlic, maple syrup, lemon zest, basil, oregano, thyme, sage, salt, black pepper, and red pepper flakes, if desired. Add the tofu and mix gently. Put in the refrigerator and marinate for 30 minutes, or up to overnight if you desire.
2.   **Cooking.** Preheat the oven to 425°F. Line a baking sheet with parchment paper or foil. Arrange the marinated tofu in a single layer on the prepared baking sheet. Bake for 20 to 30 minutes, turning over halfway through, until slightly crispy on the outside and tender on the inside.

Parmesan Zucchini Sticks

PREP TIME: 10 MINUTES / COOK TIME: 20 MINUTES/ SERVES 4
Ingredients
4 zucchini, quartered lengthwise
2 tablespoons extra-virgin olive oil
½ cup (4 ounces) grated Parmesan cheese
1 tablespoon Italian seasoning
½ teaspoon sea salt
¼ teaspoon garlic powder
⅛ teaspoon freshly ground black pepper

Directions
1.   **Preparing the Ingredients**
Preheat the oven to 350°F. In a large bowl, toss the zucchini with the olive oil.
In a small bowl, whisk the cheese, Italian seasoning, sea salt, garlic powder, and pepper. Toss with the zucchini.
Place the zucchini in a single layer on a rimmed baking sheet.
2.   **Cooking.** Bake for 15 to 20 minutes until the zucchini is soft.
Set the oven to broil, and broil for 1 to 2 minutes until the cheese-herb coating crisps, watching carefully so it doesn't burn.

Moroccan-Inspired Chickpea Tagine

PREP TIME: 20 MINUTES / COOK TIME: 40 MINUTES/ SERVES 2 WITH LEFTOVERS FOR LUNCH
Ingredients
2 tablespoons olive oil
½ onion, diced
1 garlic clove, minced
2 cups cauliflower florets
1 cup diced eggplant (large dice)
1 medium carrot, cut into 1-inch pieces
2 small red potatoes, cut into 1-inch pieces
1 (28-ounce) can whole tomatoes with their juices
1 (15-ounce) can chickpeas, drained and rinsed
1 cup water
1 teaspoon sugar
1 teaspoon cumin
½ teaspoon turmeric
½ teaspoon cinnamon
½ teaspoon salt
1 to 2 teaspoons harissa paste

Directions
Preparing the Ingredients
1.   Heat the olive oil in a Dutch oven over medium-high heat. Add the onion and sauté for 5 minutes.
2.   Add the garlic, cauliflower, eggplant, carrot, potatoes, and tomatoes. Stir, breaking up the tomatoes with a spatula. Add the chickpeas, water, sugar, cumin, turmeric, cinnamon, and salt.
Bring the mixture to a boil, and then reduce the heat to medium-low. Add 1 teaspoon of the harissa. Taste and add another 1 teaspoon if you prefer the stew spicier.
3.   Cover the pot and let the stew simmer for about 40 minutes, or until the vegetables are tender. Taste and add additional salt and any other spices, if needed.

Green beans with Potatoes and Basil (Instant Pot)

PREP TIME: 30 MINUTES / COOK TIME: 30 MINUTES/ SERVES 4
Ingredients
2 tablespoons extra-virgin olive oil, plus extra for drizzling
1 onion, chopped fine
2 tablespoons minced fresh oregano or 2 teaspoons dried
2 tablespoons tomato paste
4 garlic cloves, minced
1 (14.5-ounce) can whole peeled tomatoes, drained with juice reserved, chopped
1 cup water
1 teaspoon table salt
¼ teaspoon pepper
1½ pounds green beans, trimmed and cut into 2-inch lengths
1pound Yukon Gold potatoes, peeled and cut into 1-inch pieces
3 tablespoons chopped fresh basil or parsley
2 tablespoons toasted pine nuts
Shaved Parmesan cheese
Directions
Preparing the Ingredients
1.   Using highest sauté function, heat oil in Instant Pot until shimmering. Add onion and cook until softened, about 5 minutes. Stir in oregano, tomato paste, and garlic and cook until fragrant, about 30 seconds. Stir in tomatoes and their juice, water, salt, and pepper, then stir in green beans and potatoes. Lock lid in place and close pressure release valve. Select high pressure cook function and cook for 5 minutes.
2.   Turn off Instant Pot and quick-release pressure. Carefully remove lid, allowing steam to escape away from you. Season with salt and pepper to taste. Sprinkle individual portions with basil, pine nuts, and Parmesan and drizzle with extra oil.

Stuffed Tomatoes with Tabbouleh

PREP TIME: 10 MINUTES / COOK TIME: 20 MINUTES/ SERVES 4
Ingredients
8 medium beefsteak or similar tomatoes
3 tablespoons extra-virgin olive oil, divided
½ cup water
½ cup uncooked regular or whole-wheat couscous
1½ cups minced fresh curly parsley (about 1 large bunch)
⅓ cup minced fresh mint
2 scallions, green and white parts, chopped (about 2 tablespoons)
¼ teaspoon freshly ground black pepper
¼ teaspoon kosher or sea salt
1 medium lemon
4 teaspoons honey
⅓ cup chopped almonds
Directions
1.   **Preparing the Ingredients**
Preheat the oven to 400°F. Slice the top off each tomato and set aside. Scoop out all the flesh inside, and put the tops, flesh, and seeds in a large mixing bowl.
2.   **Cooking**
Grease a baking dish with 1 tablespoon of oil. Place the carved-out tomatoes in the baking dish, and cover with aluminum foil. Roast for 10 minutes. While the tomatoes are cooking, make the couscous by bringing the water to boil in a medium saucepan. Pour in the couscous, remove from the heat, and cover. Let sit for 5 minutes, then stir with a fork. While the couscous is cooking, chop up the tomato flesh and tops. Drain off the excess tomato water using a colander. Measure out 1 cup of the chopped tomatoes (reserve any remaining chopped tomatoes for another use). Add the cup of tomatoes back into the mixing bowl. Mix in the parsley, mint, scallions, pepper, and salt.
Using a Microplane or citrus grater, zest the lemon into the mixing bowl. Halve the lemon, and squeeze the juice through a strainer (to catch the seeds) from both halves into the bowl with the tomato mixture. Mix well.
When the couscous is ready, add it to the tomato mixture and mix well. With oven mitts, carefully remove the tomatoes from the oven. Divide the tabbouleh evenly among the tomatoes and stuff them, using a spoon to press the filling down so it all fits. Cover the pan with the foil and return it to the oven. Cook for another 8 to 10 minutes, or until the tomatoes are tender-firm. (If you prefer softer tomatoes, roast for an additional 10 minutes.) Before serving, top each tomato with a drizzle of ½ teaspoon of honey and about 2 teaspoons of almonds.

Ricotta, Basil, and Pistachio–Stuffed Zucchini

PREP TIME: 15 MINUTES / COOK TIME: 25 MINUTES/ SERVES 4
Ingredients

2 medium zucchini, halved lengthwise
1 tablespoon extra-virgin olive oil
1 onion, diced
1 teaspoon kosher salt
2 garlic cloves, minced
¾ cup ricotta cheese
¼ cup unsalted pistachios, shelled and chopped
¼ cup fresh basil, chopped
1 large egg, beaten
¼ teaspoon freshly ground black pepper
Directions
1.   Preparing the Ingredients
Preheat the oven to 425°F. Line a baking sheet with parchment paper or foil.
Scoop out the seeds/pulp from the zucchini, leaving ¼-inch flesh around the edges. Transfer the pulp to a cutting board and chop the pulp.
2.   Cooking
Heat the olive oil in a large skillet or sauté pan over medium heat. Add the onion, pulp, and salt and sauté about 5 minutes. Add the garlic and sauté 30 seconds. In a medium bowl, combine the ricotta cheese, pistachios, basil, egg, and black pepper. Add the onion mixture and mix together well. Place the 4 zucchini halves on the prepared baking sheet. Fill the zucchini halves with the ricotta mixture. Bake for 20 minutes, or until golden brown.

Lemon Kale with Slivered Almonds

PREP TIME: 10 MINUTES / COOK TIME: 10 MINUTES/ SERVES 4
Ingredients
2 tablespoons extra-virgin olive oil
4 cups chopped stemmed kale
½ teaspoon sea salt
⅛ teaspoon freshly ground black pepper
Juice of 1 lemon
Zest of 1 lemon
¼ cup slivered almonds
Directions
Preparing the Ingredients
1.   In a large skillet over medium-high heat, heat the olive oil until it shimmers.
Add the kale, sea salt, and pepper. Cook for 7 to 10 minutes, stirring occasionally, until soft.
2.   Add the lemon juice and zest and the almonds. Cook for about 3 minutes more, stirring occasionally, until the liquid reduces by half. Serve immediately.

Sautéed Cabbage with Parsley and Lemon

PREP TIME: 10 MINUTES / COOK TIME: 10 MINUTES/ SERVES 4 TO 6
Ingredients
1 small head green cabbage (1¼ pounds), cored and sliced thin
2 tablespoons extra-virgin olive oil
1 onion, halved and sliced thin
Salt and pepper
¼ cup chopped fresh parsley

1½ teaspoons lemon juice
Directions
1.   Preparing the Ingredients
Place cabbage in large bowl and cover with cold water. Let sit for 3 minutes; drain well.
2.   Cooking
Heat 1 tablespoon oil in 12-inch nonstick skillet over medium-high heat until shimmering. Add onion and ¼ teaspoon salt and cook until softened and lightly browned, 5 to 7 minutes; transfer to bowl.
Heat remaining 1 tablespoon oil in now-empty skillet over medium-high heat until shimmering. Add cabbage and sprinkle with ½ teaspoon salt and ¼ teaspoon pepper. Cover and cook, without stirring, until cabbage is wilted and lightly browned on bottom, about 3 minutes. Stir and continue to cook, uncovered, until cabbage is crisp-tender and lightly browned in places, about 4 minutes, stirring once halfway through cooking. Off heat, stir in onion, parsley, and lemon juice. Season with salt and pepper to taste and serve.

Braised Radishes with Sugar Snap Peas and Dukkah (Instant Pot)

PREP TIME: 22 MINUTES / COOK TIME: 2 MINUTES/ SERVES 4
Ingredients
¼ cup extra-virgin olive oil, divided
1 shallot, sliced thin
3 garlic cloves, sliced thin
1½ pounds radishes, 2 cups greens reserved, radishes trimmed and halved if small or quartered if large
½ cup water
½ teaspoon table salt
8 ounces sugar snap peas, strings removed, sliced thin on bias
8 ounces cremini mushrooms, trimmed and sliced thin
2 teaspoons grated lemon zest plus 1 teaspoon juice
1 cup plain Greek yogurt
½ cup fresh cilantro leaves
3 tablespoons dukkah
Directions
Preparing the Ingredients
1.   Using highest sauté function, heat 2 tablespoons oil in Instant Pot until shimmering. Add shallot and cook until softened, about 2 minutes. Stir in garlic and cook until fragrant, about 30 seconds. Stir in radishes, water, and salt.
2.   Lock lid in place and close pressure release valve. Select high pressure cook function and cook for 1 minute.
3.   Turn off Instant Pot and quick-release pressure. Carefully remove lid, allowing steam to escape away from you. Stir in snap peas, cover, and let sit until heated through, about 3 minutes. Add radish greens, mushrooms, lemon zest and juice, and remaining 2 tablespoons oil and gently toss to combine. Season with salt and pepper to taste.

4. Spread ¼ cup yogurt over bottom of 4 individual serving plates. Using slotted spoon, arrange vegetable mixture on top and sprinkle with cilantro and dukkah. Serve.

Farro with Roasted Tomatoes and Mushrooms

PREP TIME: 20 MINUTES / COOK TIME: 1 HOUR/ SERVES 4- 6

Ingredients

2 pints cherry tomatoes
1 teaspoon extra-virgin olive oil
¼ teaspoon kosher salt
3 to 4 cups water
½ cup farro
¼ teaspoon kosher salt
2 tablespoons extra-virgin olive oil
1 onion, julienned
½ teaspoon kosher salt
¼ teaspoon freshly ground black pepper
10 ounces baby bella (crimini) mushrooms, stemmed and sliced thin
½ cup no-salt-added vegetable stock
1 (15-ounce) can no-salt-added or low-sodium cannellini beans, drained and rinsed
1 cup baby spinach
2 tablespoons fresh basil, cut into ribbons
¼ cup pine nuts, toasted
Aged balsamic vinegar (optional)

Directions

Preparing the Ingredients

1. Preheat the oven to 400°F. Line a baking sheet with parchment paper or foil. Toss the tomatoes, olive oil, and salt together on the baking sheet and roast for 30 minutes.
2. Bring the water, farro, and salt to a boil in a medium saucepan or pot over high heat. Cover, reduce the heat to low, and simmer, and cook for 30 minutes, or until the farro is al dente. Drain and set aside.
3. Heat the olive oil in a large skillet or sauté pan over medium-low heat. Add the onions, salt, and black pepper and sauté until golden brown and starting to caramelize, about 15 minutes. Add the mushrooms, increase the heat to medium, and sauté until the liquid has evaporated and the mushrooms brown, about 10 minutes.
Add the vegetable stock and deglaze the pan, scraping up any brown bits, and reduce the liquid for about 5 minutes. Add the beans and warm through, about 3 minutes. Remove from the heat and mix in the spinach, basil, pine nuts, roasted tomatoes, and farro. Garnish with a drizzle of balsamic vinegar, if desired.

Roasted Fennel with Tomatoes

PREP TIME: 10 MINUTES / COOK TIME: 25 MINUTES/ SERVES 4

Ingredients

2 fennel bulbs, cored and cut into ½-inch-thick pieces
20 cherry tomatoes, halved
¼ cup extra-virgin olive oil
½ teaspoon sea salt
¼ teaspoon freshly ground black pepper

Directions

1. **Preparing the Ingredients**
Preheat the oven to 425°F. In a large bowl, toss the fennel and tomatoes with the olive oil, sea salt, and pepper. Spread in an even layer in a roasting pan or on a rimmed baking sheet.
2. **Cooking**
Roast for 20 to 25 minutes until the fennel is soft and browned. Serve hot. Add ¼ cup pine nuts to the vegetables before roasting.

One-Pan Mushroom Pasta with Mascarpone

PREP TIME: 10 MINUTES / COOK TIME: 20 MINUTES/ SERVES 2

Ingredients

2 tablespoons olive oil
1 large shallot, minced
8 ounces baby bella (cremini) mushrooms, sliced
¼ cup dry sherry
1 teaspoon dried thyme
2 cups low-sodium vegetable stock
6 ounces dry pappardelle pasta
2 tablespoons mascarpone cheese
Salt
Freshly ground black pepper

Directions

Preparing the Ingredients

1. Heat olive oil in a large sauté pan over medium-high heat.
Add the shallot and mushrooms and sauté for 10 minutes, or until the mushrooms have given up much of their liquid. Add the sherry, thyme, and vegetable stock. Bring the mixture to a boil. Add the pasta, breaking it up as needed so it fits into the pan and is covered by the liquid. Return the mixture to a boil. Cover, and reduce the heat to medium-low. Let the pasta cook for 10 minutes, or until al dente.
Stir it occasionally so it doesn't stick. If the sauce gets too dry, add some water or additional chicken stock.
2. When the pasta is tender, stir in the mascarpone cheese and season with salt and pepper. The sauce will thicken up a bit when it's off the heat.

Spiced Winter Squash with Halloumi and Shaved Brussels Sprouts

PREP TIME: 30 MINUTES / COOK TIME: 30 MINUTES/ SERVES 4

Ingredients

3 tablespoons extra-virgin olive oil, divided
2 tablespoons lemon juice
2 garlic cloves, minced, divided
⅛ teaspoon plus ½ teaspoon table salt, divided
8 ounces Brussels sprouts, trimmed, halved, and sliced very thin

1 (8-ounce) block halloumi cheese, sliced crosswise into ¾-inch-thick slabs
4 scallions, white parts minced, green parts sliced thin on bias
½ teaspoon ground cardamom
¼ teaspoon ground cumin
⅛ teaspoon cayenne pepper
2 pounds butternut squash, peeled, seeded, and cut into 1-inch pieces (5 cups)
½ cup chicken or vegetable broth
2 teaspoons honey
¼ cup dried cherries
2 tablespoons roasted pepitas

Directions

1.   Preparing the Ingredients
Whisk 1 tablespoon oil, lemon juice, ¼ teaspoon garlic, and ⅛ teaspoon salt together in bowl. Add Brussels sprouts and toss to coat; let sit until ready to serve.

2.   Cooking
Using highest sauté function, heat remaining 2 tablespoons oil in Instant Pot until shimmering. Arrange halloumi around edges of pot and cook until browned, about 3 minutes per side; transfer to plate. Add scallion whites to fat left in pot and cook until softened, about 2 minutes. Stir in remaining garlic, cardamom, cumin, and cayenne and cook until fragrant, about 30 seconds. Stir in squash, broth, and remaining ½ teaspoon salt. Lock lid in place and close pressure release valve. Select high pressure cook function and cook for 6 minutes.

Turn off Instant Pot and quick-release pressure. Carefully remove lid, allowing steam to escape away from you. Using highest sauté function, continue to cook squash mixture, stirring occasionally until liquid is almost completely evaporated, about 5 minutes. Turn off Instant Pot. Using potato masher, mash squash until mostly smooth. Season with salt and pepper to taste.

Spread portion of squash over bottom of individual serving plates. Top with Brussels sprouts and halloumi. Drizzle with honey and sprinkle with cherries, pepitas, and scallion greens.

North African Peanut Stew Over Cauliflower Rice

PREP TIME: 5 MINUTES / COOK TIME: 25 MINUTES/ SERVES 4

Ingredients
1 cup frozen corn
2 tablespoons extra-virgin olive oil
1 cup chopped onion (about ½ medium onion)
2 medium Yukon Gold potatoes, unpeeled, cut into ½-inch cubes (about 2 cups)
1 large sweet potato, unpeeled, cut into ½-inch cubes (about 2 cups)
3 garlic cloves, minced (about 1½ teaspoons)
1½ teaspoons ground cumin
1 teaspoon ground allspice

1 teaspoon freshly grated ginger root or ½ teaspoon ground ginger
½ teaspoon crushed red pepper, or to taste
¼ teaspoon kosher or sea salt
½ cup water
1 (28-ounce) can diced tomatoes, undrained
1 (12-ounce) package frozen plain cauliflower rice
1 (15-ounce) can lentils, undrained
⅓ cup creamy peanut butter
Pickled hot peppers, chopped roasted peanuts, chopped fresh cilantro, for serving (optional)

Directions

1.   **Preparing the Ingredients.** Put the corn on the counter to partially thaw while making the stew.

2.   **Cooking.** In a large stockpot over medium-high heat, heat the oil. Add the onion, potatoes, and sweet potatoes. Cook for 7 minutes, stirring occasionally, until some of the potatoes and onion get golden and crispy. Move the potatoes to the edges of the pot, and add the garlic, cumin, allspice, ginger, crushed red pepper, and salt. Cook for 1 minute, stirring constantly. Stir in the water and cook for 1 more minute, scraping up the crispy bits from the bottom of the pan. Add the tomatoes with their juices to the stockpot. Cook for 15 minutes uncovered, stirring occasionally. While the tomatoes are cooking, cook the cauliflower rice according to the package directions. Into the tomato mixture, stir in the lentils, partially thawed corn, and peanut butter. Reduce the heat to medium and cook for 1 to 2 minutes, until all the ingredients are warmed, stirring constantly to blend in the peanut butter. Serve over the cauliflower rice with hot peppers, peanuts, and fresh cilantro, if desired.

Baked Orzo with Eggplant, Swiss Chard, and Mozzarella

PREP TIME: 20 MINUTES / COOK TIME: 1 HOUR/ SERVES 4- 6

Ingredients
2 tablespoons extra-virgin olive oil
1 large (1-pound) eggplant, diced small
2 carrots, peeled and diced small
2 celery stalks, diced small
1 onion, diced small
½ teaspoon kosher salt
3 garlic cloves, minced
¼ teaspoon freshly ground black pepper
1 cup whole-wheat orzo
1 teaspoon no-salt-added tomato paste
1½ cups no-salt-added vegetable stock
1 cup Swiss chard, stemmed and chopped small
2 tablespoons fresh oregano, chopped
Zest of 1 lemon
4 ounces mozzarella cheese, diced small
¼ cup grated Parmesan cheese
2 tomatoes, sliced ½-inch-thick

Directions

Preparing the Ingredients

flakes and sauté until the garlic is a light golden brown, about 2 minutes. Add the tomatoes, salt, and honey and mix well. Reduce the heat to low and simmer for 20 minutes. Add the kale and mix in well. Cook about 5 minutes. Add the chickpeas and simmer about 5 minutes.

2.   Remove from heat and stir in the basil. Serve topped with pecorino cheese.

Grilled Eggplant Stacks

PREP TIME: 20 MINUTES / COOK TIME: 10 MINUTES/ SERVES 2

Ingredients

1 medium eggplant, cut crosswise into 8 slices
¼ teaspoon salt
1 teaspoon Italian herb seasoning mix
2 tablespoons olive oil
1 large tomato, cut into 4 slices
4 (1-ounce) slices of buffalo mozzarella
Fresh basil, for garnish

Directions

1.   **Preparing the Ingredients**
Place the eggplant slices in a colander set in the sink or over a bowl. Sprinkle both sides with the salt. Let the eggplant sit for 15 minutes.
While the eggplant is resting, heat the grill to medium-high heat (about 350°F).
Pat the eggplant dry with paper towels and place it in a mixing bowl. Sprinkle it with the Italian herb seasoning mix and olive oil. Toss well to coat.

2.   **Cooking.** Grill the eggplant for 5 minutes, or until it has grill marks and is lightly charred. Flip each eggplant slice over, and grill on the second side for another 5 minutes.
Flip the eggplant slices back over and top four of the slices with a slice of tomato and a slice of mozzarella. Top each stack with one of the remaining four slices of eggplant.
Turn the grill down to low and cover it to let the cheese melt. Check after 30 seconds and remove when the cheese is soft and mostly melted.
Sprinkle with fresh basil slices.

Roasted Feta with Kale and Lemon Yogurt

PREP TIME: 15 MINUTES / COOK TIME: 20 MINUTES/ SERVES 4

Ingredients

1 tablespoon extra-virgin olive oil
1 onion, julienned
¼ teaspoon kosher salt
1 teaspoon ground turmeric
½ teaspoon ground cumin
½ teaspoon ground coriander
¼ teaspoon freshly ground black pepper
1 bunch kale, stemmed and chopped
7-ounce block feta cheese, cut into ¼-inch-thick slices
½ cup plain Greek yogurt
1 tablespoon lemon juice

Directions

1.   **Preparing the Ingredients**. Preheat the oven to 400°F. Heat the olive oil in a large ovenproof skillet or sauté pan over medium heat. Add the onion and salt; sauté until lightly golden brown, about 5 minutes. Add the turmeric, cumin, coriander, and black pepper; sauté for 30 seconds. Add the kale and sauté about 2 minutes. Add ½ cup water and continue to cook down the kale, about 3 minutes.

2.   Remove from the heat and place the feta cheese slices on top of the kale mixture. Place in the oven and bake until the feta softens, 10 to 12 minutes. In a small bowl, combine the yogurt and lemon juice. Serve the kale and feta cheese topped with the lemon yogurt.

Stuffed Red Bell Peppers

PREP TIME: 20 MINUTES / COOK TIME: 50 MINUTES/ SERVES 4

Ingredients

4 red bell peppers, tops, seeds and ribs removed
2 tablespoons extra-virgin olive oil
1 onion, finely chopped
1 zucchini, chopped
3 garlic cloves, minced
3 Roma tomatoes, chopped
4 cups fresh baby spinach
1 teaspoon dried oregano
½ teaspoon sea salt
¼ teaspoon freshly ground black pepper
1 cup cooked brown rice
4 ounces crumbled feta cheese

Directions

1.   **Preparing the Ingredients.** Preheat the oven to 350°F. Place the peppers, cut-side up, in a 9-inch-square baking pan.

2.   **Cooking.** In a large skillet over medium-high heat, heat the olive oil until it shimmers. Add the onion and zucchini. Cook for about 5 minutes, stirring occasionally, until the vegetables are soft. Add the garlic and cook for 30 seconds, stirring constantly. Add the tomatoes, spinach, oregano, sea salt, and pepper. Cook for about 3 minutes, stirring occasionally, until the spinach wilts. Remove the pan from the heat. Stir in the rice until well blended. Spoon the rice mixture into the bell peppers. Sprinkle the feta over the tops. Add about ¼ cup water to the baking pan and cover it with aluminum foil. Bake for 30 minutes. Uncover and bake for about 10 minutes more until the cheese bubbles and browns.

Asparagus and Mushroom Farrotto

PREP TIME: 20 MINUTES / COOK TIME: 45 MINUTES/ SERVES 2

Ingredients

½ ounce dried porcini mushrooms
1 cup hot water
3 cups low-sodium vegetable stock
2 tablespoons olive oil
½ large onion, minced (about 1 cup)
1 garlic clove

1 cup diced mushrooms (about 4 ounces)
¾ cup farro
½ cup dry white wine
½ teaspoon dried thyme
4 ounces asparagus, cut into ½-inch pieces (about 1 cup)
2 tablespoons grated Parmesan cheese
Salt

Directions

1. Preparing the Ingredients

Soak the dried mushrooms in the hot water for about 15 minutes. When they're softened, drain the mushrooms, reserving the liquid. Mince the porcini mushrooms. Add the mushroom liquid and vegetable stock to a medium saucepan and bring it to a boil. Reduce the heat to low just to keep it warm.

2. Cooking

Heat the olive oil in a Dutch oven over high heat. Add the onion, garlic, and mushrooms, and sauté for 10 minutes. Add the farro to the Dutch oven and sauté it for 3 minutes to toast.

Add the wine, thyme, and one ladleful of the hot mushroom and chicken stock.

Bring it to a boil while stirring the farro. Do not cover the pot while the farro is cooking. Reduce the heat to medium. When the liquid is absorbed, add another ladleful or two at a time to the pot, stirring occasionally, until the farro is cooked through. Keep an eye on the heat, to make sure it doesn't cook too quickly. When the farro is al dente, add the asparagus and another ladleful of stock.

Cook for another 3 to 5 minutes, or until the asparagus is softened. Stir in Parmesan cheese and season with salt.

Roasted Eggplant and Chickpeas with Tomato Sauce

PREP TIME: 15 MINUTES / COOK TIME: 1 HOUR/ SERVES 4

Ingredients

Olive oil cooking spray
1 large (about 1 pound) eggplant, sliced into ¼-inch-thick rounds
1 teaspoon kosher salt, divided
1 tablespoon extra-virgin olive oil
3 garlic cloves, minced
1 (28-ounce) can no-salt-added crushed tomatoes
½ teaspoon honey
¼ teaspoon freshly ground black pepper
2 tablespoons fresh basil, chopped
1 (15-ounce) can no-salt-added or low-sodium chickpeas, drained and rinsed
¾ cup crumbled feta cheese
1 tablespoon fresh oregano, chopped

Directions

1. Preparing the Ingredients

Preheat the oven to 425°F. Line two baking sheets with foil and lightly spray with olive oil cooking spray. Arrange the eggplant in a single layer and sprinkle with ½ teaspoon of the salt.

2. Cooking

Bake for 20 minutes, turning once halfway, until lightly golden brown. Meanwhile, heat the olive oil in a large saucepan over medium heat. Add the garlic and sauté for 30 seconds. Add the crushed tomatoes, honey, the remaining ½ teaspoon salt, and black pepper. Simmer about 20 minutes, until the sauce reduces a bit and thickens. Stir in the basil. After removing the eggplant from the oven, reduce the oven temperature to 375°F. In a large rectangular or oval baking dish, ladle in the chickpeas and 1 cup sauce. Layer the eggplant slices on top, overlapping as necessary to cover the chickpeas. Spread the remaining sauce on top of the eggplant. Sprinkle the feta cheese and oregano on top.

Cover the baking dish with foil and bake for 15 minutes. Remove the foil and bake an additional 15 minutes.

Baked Stuffed Portobello Mushrooms

PREP TIME: 20 MINUTES / COOK TIME: 45 MINUTES/ SERVES 4

Ingredients

4 portobello mushrooms, stems and gills removed
2 tablespoons extra-virgin olive oil
1 onion, finely chopped
1 zucchini, chopped
1 red bell pepper, chopped
2 cups kale
½ teaspoon sea salt
¼ teaspoon freshly ground black pepper
⅛ teaspoon red pepper flakes
4 garlic cloves, minced
¼ cup chopped fresh basil leaves
4 ounces grated part-skim mozzarella

Directions

1. Preparing the Ingredients

Preheat the oven to 350°F. Place the mushrooms, gill-side up, on a rimmed baking sheet.

In a large skillet over medium-high heat, heat the olive oil until it shimmers.

2. Cooking

Add the onion, zucchini, red bell pepper, kale, sea salt, pepper, and red pepper flakes. Cook for about 5 minutes, stirring occasionally, until the vegetables are soft. Add the garlic and cook for 30 seconds, stirring constantly. Remove the pan from the heat. Stir in the basil. Spoon the vegetable mixture into the mushroom caps.

Sprinkle the cheese over the tops. Bake for 30 to 40 minutes until the cheese is brown and bubbly and the mushrooms are soft.

Sheet Pan Roasted Chickpeas and Vegetables with Harissa Yogurt

PREP TIME: 10 MINUTES / COOK TIME: 30 MINUTES/ SERVES 2

Ingredients

4 cups cauliflower florets (about ½ small head)

2 medium carrots, peeled, halved, and then sliced into quarters lengthwise
2 tablespoons olive oil, divided
½ teaspoon garlic powder, divided
½ teaspoon salt, divided
2 teaspoons za'atar spice mix, divided
1 (15-ounce) can chickpeas, drained, rinsed, and patted dry
¾ cup plain Greek yogurt
1 teaspoon harissa spice paste
Directions
1.   Preparing the Ingredients
Preheat the oven to 400°F and set the rack to the middle position. Line a sheet pan with foil or parchment paper. Place the cauliflower and carrots in a large bowl. Drizzle with 1 tablespoon olive oil and sprinkle with ¼ teaspoon of garlic powder, ¼ teaspoon of salt, and 1 teaspoon of za'atar. Toss well to combine. Spread the vegetables onto one half of the sheet pan in a single layer. Place the chickpeas in the same bowl and season with the remaining 1 tablespoon of oil, ¼ teaspoon of garlic powder, and ¼ teaspoon of salt, and the remaining za'atar. Toss well to combine. Spread the chickpeas onto the other half of the sheet pan.
2.   Cooking
Roast for 30 minutes, or until the vegetables are tender and the chickpeas start to turn golden. Flip the vegetables halfway through the cooking time, and give the chickpeas a stir so they cook evenly. The chickpeas may need an extra few minutes if you like them crispy. If so, remove the vegetables and leave the chickpeas in until they're cooked to desired crispiness.
While the vegetables are roasting, combine the yogurt and harissa in a small bowl. Taste, and add additional harissa as desired.

Baked Falafel Sliders

PREP TIME: 10 MINUTES / COOK TIME: 30 MINUTES/ MAKES: 6 SLIDERS
Ingredients
Olive oil cooking spray
1 (15-ounce) can no-salt-added or low-sodium chickpeas, drained and rinsed
1 onion, roughly chopped
2 garlic cloves, peeled
2 tablespoons fresh parsley, chopped
2 tablespoons whole-wheat flour
½ teaspoon ground coriander
½ teaspoon ground cumin
½ teaspoon baking powder
½ teaspoon kosher salt
¼ teaspoon freshly ground black pepper
Directions
1.   Preparing the Ingredients
Preheat the oven to 350°F. Line a baking sheet with parchment paper or foil and lightly spray with olive oil cooking spray. In a food processor, add the chickpeas, onion, garlic, parsley, flour, coriander,

cumin, baking powder, salt, and black pepper. Process until smooth, stopping to scrape down the sides of the bowl.
2.   Cooking
Make 6 slider patties, each with a heaping ¼ cup of mixture, and arrange on the prepared baking sheet. Bake for 30 minutes, turning over halfway through.

Falafel Patties

PREP TIME: 15 MINUTES (PLUS 24 HOURS TO REST) / COOK TIME: 30 MINUTES/ SERVES 8
Ingredients
1 cup dried chickpeas
1 red onion, minced, divided
2 tablespoons chopped fresh cilantro leaves
4 garlic cloves, minced
1 teaspoon dried cumin
1 tablespoon freshly squeezed lemon juice
1 teaspoon sea salt
1 teaspoon baking powder
3 tablespoons extra-virgin olive oil
1 tomato, chopped
¼ cup chopped fresh Italian parsley leaves
Directions
1.   Preparing the Ingredients
In a large bowl, combine the chickpeas with enough water to cover. Cover the bowl and let sit at room temperature for 24 hours to soak. Add more water as needed to keep the chickpeas covered. Drain thoroughly. Preheat the oven to 375°F. Line a baking sheet with parchment paper or aluminum foil. In a food processor, combine the chickpeas, all but 2 tablespoons of the red onion, the cilantro, garlic, cumin, lemon juice, sea salt, and baking powder. Pulse for 10 to 20 (1-second) pulses until the ingredients are finely chopped but not puréed. Form the mixture into 8 patties.
2.   Cooking
Brush the patties with olive oil on both sides and place them on the prepared sheet. Bake for 10 to 15 minutes, flip, and bake for 10 to 15 minutes more until each side is golden brown. Garnish with the reserved 2 tablespoons of red onion, the tomato, and parsley.

Quinoa Lentil "Meatballs" With Quick Tomato Sauce

PREP TIME: 25 MINUTES / COOK TIME: 45 MINUTES/ SERVES 4
Ingredients
Olive oil cooking spray
2 large eggs, beaten
1 tablespoon no-salt-added tomato paste
½ teaspoon kosher salt
½ cup grated Parmesan cheese
½ onion, roughly chopped
¼ cup fresh parsley
1 garlic clove, peeled
1½ cups cooked lentils
1 cup cooked quinoa

1 tablespoon extra-virgin olive oil
1 onion, minced
½ teaspoon dried oregano
½ teaspoon kosher salt
2 garlic cloves, minced
1 (28-ounce) can no-salt-added crushed tomatoes
½ teaspoon honey
¼ cup fresh basil, chopped
Directions
1.   Preparing the Ingredients
Preheat the oven to 400°F. Lightly grease a 12-cup muffin pan with olive oil cooking spray.
In a large bowl, whisk together the eggs, tomato paste, and salt until fully combined. Mix in the Parmesan cheese. In a food processor, add the onion, parsley, and garlic. Process until minced.
Add to the egg mixture and stir together. Add the lentils to the food processor and process until puréed into a thick paste. Add to the large bowl and mix together. Add the quinoa and mix well. Form balls, slightly larger than a golf ball, with ¼ cup of the quinoa mixture. Place each ball in a muffin pan cup. Note: The mixture will be somewhat soft but should hold together.
2.   Cooking
Bake 25 to 30 minutes, until golden brown. To make the tomato sauce
Heat the olive oil in a large saucepan over medium heat. Add the onion, oregano, and salt and sauté until light golden brown, about 5 minutes. Add the garlic and cook for 30 seconds.
Stir in the tomatoes and honey.
Increase the heat to high and cook, stirring often, until simmering, then decrease the heat to medium-low and cook for 10 minutes. Remove from the heat and stir in the basil. Serve with the meatballs.

Broiled Eggplant with Basil
PREP TIME: 10 MINUTES / COOK TIME: 8 MINUTES/ SERVES 4 TO 6
Ingredients
1½ pounds eggplant, sliced into ¼-inch-thick rounds
Kosher salt and pepper
3 tablespoons extra-virgin olive oil
2 tablespoons chopped fresh basil
Directions
1.   Preparing the Ingredients
Spread eggplant on paper towel–lined baking sheet, sprinkle both sides with 1½ teaspoons salt, and let sit for 30 minutes.
2.   Cooking
Adjust oven rack 4 inches from broiler element and heat broiler. Thoroughly pat eggplant dry with paper towels, arrange on aluminum foil–lined rimmed baking sheet in single layer, and brush both sides with oil. Broil eggplant until mahogany brown and lightly charred, about 4 minutes per side. Transfer eggplant to serving platter, season with pepper to taste, and sprinkle with basil. Serve.

Three-Bean Vegetable Chili
PREP TIME: 20 MINUTES / COOK TIME: 20 MINUTES/ SERVES 8
Ingredients
2 tablespoons extra-virgin olive oil
2 green bell peppers, seeded and chopped
1 onion, chopped
6 garlic cloves, minced
1 (14-ounce) can kidney beans, drained
1 (14-ounce) can black beans, drained
1 (14-ounce) can pinto beans, drained
2 (14-ounce) cans crushed tomatoes
1 tablespoon chili powder
1 teaspoon ground cumin
1 teaspoon sea salt
¼ teaspoon cayenne pepper
Directions
Preparing the Ingredients
In a large pot over medium-high heat, heat the olive oil until it shimmers. Add the green bell peppers and onion. Cook for about 5 minutes, stirring occasionally, until soft. Add the garlic and cook for 30 seconds, stirring constantly.
Stir in the kidney beans, black beans, pinto beans, tomatoes, chili powder, cumin, sea salt, and cayenne. Bring to a simmer. Reduce the heat to medium-low and cook for 10 minutes more, stirring occasionally. Remove from the heat and serve.

Spaghetti Squash Marinara
PREP TIME: 20 MINUTES / COOK TIME: 45 MINUTES/ SERVES 4
Ingredients
1 spaghetti squash, halved lengthwise and seeded
2 tablespoons extra-virgin olive oil
1 onion, chopped
6 garlic cloves, minced
2 (14-ounce) cans crushed tomatoes
1 (14-ounce) can chopped tomatoes, drained
1 tablespoon dried Italian seasoning
1 teaspoon dried oregano
½ teaspoon sea salt
¼ teaspoon red pepper flakes
Directions
Preparing the Ingredients
**1.   **Preheat the oven to 375°F. Place the squash, cut-side down, on a rimmed baking sheet. Bake for about 45 minutes until soft. While the squash cooks, in a large pot over medium-high heat, heat the olive oil until it shimmers. Add the onion. Cook for about 5 minutes, stirring occasionally, until soft. Add the garlic and cook for 30 seconds, stirring constantly.
**2.   **Stir in the crushed and chopped tomatoes, Italian seasoning, oregano, sea salt, and red pepper flakes.
Bring to a simmer and reduce the heat to medium-low. Simmer for 10 minutes, stirring occasionally. Once the squash is cooked, let it cool slightly before handling.

Using a fork, scrape the flesh away from the rind into spaghetti-like noodles and place in a serving bowl. Spoon the sauce over the squash and serve.

3.		To make the squash in a slow cooker, leave it whole and uncut. Prick the rind all over with a fork and place it in the cooker.

Cook for 8 hours on low. No additional liquid is required, because the squash releases its own moisture.

When done cooking, halve the squash and use a fork to scrape the flesh into strands.

Braised Fennel with Radicchio and Parmesan

PREP TIME: 10 MINUTES / COOK TIME: 30 MINUTES/ SERVES 6

Ingredients

3 tablespoons extra-virgin olive oil
3 fennel bulbs (12 ounces each), 2 tablespoons fronds minced, stalks discarded, bulbs cut vertically into ½-inch-thick slabs
½ teaspoon grated lemon zest plus 2 teaspoons juice
Salt and pepper
½ cup dry white wine
1 head radicchio (10 ounces), cored and sliced thin
¼ cup water
2 teaspoons honey
2 tablespoons pine nuts, toasted and chopped
Shaved Parmesan cheese

Directions

Preparing the Ingredients

1.		Heat oil in 12-inch skillet over medium heat until shimmering. Add fennel pieces, lemon zest, ½ teaspoon salt, and ¼ teaspoon pepper, then pour wine over fennel. (Skillet will be slightly crowded at first, but fennel will fit into single layer as it cooks.) Cover, reduce heat to medium-low, and cook until fennel is just tender, about 20 minutes.

2.		Increase heat to medium, flip fennel pieces, and continue to cook, uncovered, until fennel is well browned on first side and liquid is almost completely evaporated, 5 to 8 minutes.

3.		Flip fennel pieces and continue to cook until well browned on second side, 2 to 4 minutes. Transfer fennel to serving platter and tent loosely with aluminum foil.

4.		Add radicchio, water, honey, and pinch salt to now-empty skillet and cook over low heat, scraping up any browned bits, until wilted, 3 to 5 minutes. Off heat, stir in lemon juice and season with salt and pepper to taste. Arrange radicchio over fennel and sprinkle with pine nuts, minced fennel fronds, and shaved Parmesan.

Zucchini Noodles with Peas and Mint

PREP TIME: 10 MINUTES / COOK TIME: 15 MINUTES/ SERVES 6

Ingredients

5 tablespoons extra-virgin olive oil, divided
1 shallot, minced
3 cups peas (fresh or frozen)
6 garlic cloves, minced
6 zucchini, spiralized into noodles
Juice of 1 lemon
Zest of 1 lemon
½ teaspoon sea salt
⅛ teaspoon freshly ground black pepper
¼ cup chopped fresh mint leaves

Directions

Preparing the Ingredients

1.		In a large pot over medium-high heat, heat 3 tablespoons of olive oil until it shimmers. Add the shallot. Cook for about 5 minutes, stirring occasionally, until soft. Add the peas. Cook for 4 minutes, stirring occasionally. Add the garlic and cook for 30 seconds, stirring constantly. Add the zucchini, lemon juice and zest, sea salt, and pepper. Cook for about 4 minutes more, stirring, until the zucchini is al dente.

2.		Toss with the remaining 2 tablespoons of olive oil and mint before serving.

FISH AND SEAFOOD MAINS

Pistachio-Crusted Whitefish

PREP TIME: 10 MINUTES / COOK TIME: 20 MINUTES / SERVES 2

Ingredients

¼ cup shelled pistachios
1 tablespoon fresh parsley
1 tablespoon grated Parmesan cheese
1 tablespoon panko bread crumbs
2 tablespoons olive oil
¼ teaspoon salt
10 ounces skinless whitefish (1 large piece or 2 smaller ones)

Directions

1.   Preparing the Ingredients

Preheat the oven to 350°F and set the rack to the middle position. Line a sheet pan with foil or parchment paper.

Combine all of the ingredients except the fish in a mini food processor, and pulse until the nuts are finely ground. Alternatively, you can mince the nuts with a chef's knife and combine the ingredients by hand in a small bowl.

Place the fish on the sheet pan.

Spread the nut mixture evenly over the fish and pat it down lightly.

2.   Cooking

Bake the fish for 20 to 30 minutes, depending on the thickness, until it flakes easily with a fork.

Keep in mind that a thicker cut of fish takes a bit longer to bake. You'll know it's done when it's opaque, flakes apart easily with a fork, or reaches an internal temperature of 145°F.

Poached Salmon (Instant Pot)

PREP TIME: 15 MINUTES / COOK TIME: 3 MINUTES / SERVES 4

Ingredients

1 lemon, sliced ¼ inch thick
4 (6-ounce) skinless salmon fillets, 1½ inches thick
½ teaspoon table salt
¼ teaspoon pepper

Directions

Preparing the Ingredients

1.   Add ½ cup water to Instant Pot. Fold sheet of aluminum foil into 16 by 6-inch sling. Arrange lemon slices widthwise in 2 rows across center of sling. Sprinkle flesh side of salmon with salt and pepper, then arrange skinned side down on top of lemon slices.

2.   Using sling, lower salmon into Instant Pot; allow narrow edges of sling to rest along sides of insert. Lock lid in place and close pressure release valve. Select high pressure cook function and cook for 3 minutes.

3.   Turn off Instant Pot and quick-release pressure. Carefully remove lid, allowing steam to escape away from you. Using sling, transfer salmon to large plate. Gently lift and tilt fillets with spatula to remove lemon slices.

Citrus-Glazed Salmon with Zucchini Noodles

PREP TIME: 10 MINUTES / COOK TIME: 20 MINUTES / SERVES 4

Ingredients

4 (5- to 6-ounce) pieces salmon
½ teaspoon kosher salt
¼ teaspoon freshly ground black pepper
1 tablespoon extra-virgin olive oil
1 cup freshly squeezed orange juice
1 teaspoon low-sodium soy sauce
2 zucchini (about 16 ounces), spiralized
1 tablespoon fresh chives, chopped
1 tablespoon fresh parsley, chopped

Directions

1.   Preparing the Ingredients

Preheat the oven to 350°F. Season the salmon with salt and black pepper.

2.   Cooking

Heat the olive oil in a large oven-safe skillet or sauté pan over medium-high heat. Add the salmon, skin-side down, and sear for 5 minutes, or until the skin is golden brown and crispy. Turn the salmon over and transfer to the oven until your desired doneness is reached—about 5 minutes for medium-rare, 7 minutes for medium, and 9 minutes for medium-well. Place the salmon on a cutting board to rest.

Place the same pan on the stove over medium-high heat.

Add the orange juice and soy sauce to deglaze the pan. Bring to a simmer, scraping up any brown bits, and continue to simmer 5 to 7 minutes, until the liquid is reduced by half to a syrup-like consistency. Divide the zucchini noodles among 4 plates and place 1 piece of salmon on each. Pour the orange glaze over the salmon and zucchini noodles. Garnish with the chives and parsley.

Shrimp Scampi

PREP TIME: 10 MINUTES / COOK TIME: 15 MINUTES/ SERVES 4

Ingredients

2 tablespoons extra-virgin olive oil
1 shallot, minced
1 pound medium shrimp, peeled, deveined, and tails removed
6 garlic cloves, minced
Juice of 1 lemon
Zest of 1 lemon
½ cup dry white wine
½ teaspoon sea salt
¼ teaspoon freshly ground black pepper
Pinch red pepper flakes
¼ cup chopped fresh Italian parsley leaves

6 ounces whole-wheat pasta, cooked according to package directions

Directions

Preparing the Ingredients

In a large skillet over medium-high heat, heat the olive oil until it shimmers. Add the shallot. Cook for about 5 minutes, stirring occasionally, until soft. Toss in the shrimp. Cook for 3 to 4 minutes, stirring occasionally, until the shrimp is pink. Add the garlic and cook for 30 seconds, stirring constantly. Stir in the lemon juice and zest, wine, sea salt, pepper, and red pepper flakes. Bring to a simmer and reduce the heat to medium-low.

Cook for about 2 minutes until the liquid reduces by half. Remove from the heat and stir in the parsley.Toss with the hot pasta and serve.

Salmon with Lemon-Garlic Mashed Cauliflower (Instant Pot)

PREP TIME: 30 MINUTES / COOK TIME: 3 MINUTES / SERVES 4

Ingredients

2 tablespoons extra-virgin olive oil
4 garlic cloves, peeled and smashed
½ cup chicken or vegetable broth
¾ teaspoon table salt, divided
1 large head cauliflower (3 pounds), cored and cut into 2-inch florets
4 (6-ounce) skinless salmon fillets, 1½ inches thick
½ teaspoon ras el hanout
½ teaspoon grated lemon zest
3 scallions, sliced thin
1 tablespoon sesame seeds, toasted

Directions

Preparing the Ingredients

Using highest sauté function, cook oil and garlic in Instant Pot until garlic is fragrant and light golden brown, about 3 minutes. Turn off Instant Pot, then stir in broth and ¼ teaspoon salt. Arrange cauliflower in pot in even layer. Fold sheet of aluminum foil into 16 by 6-inch sling. Sprinkle flesh side of salmon with ras el hanout and remaining ½ teaspoon salt, then arrange skinned side down in center of sling. Using sling, lower salmon into Instant Pot on top of cauliflower; allow narrow edges of sling to rest along sides of insert.

Lock lid in place and close pressure release valve. Select high pressure cook function and cook for 2 minutes. Turn off Instant Pot and quick-release pressure. Carefully remove lid, allowing steam to escape away from you. Using sling, transfer salmon to large plate. Tent with foil and let rest while finishing cauliflower.

Using potato masher, mash cauliflower mixture until no large chunks remain.

Using highest sauté function, cook cauliflower, stirring often, until slightly thickened, about 3 minutes. Stir in lemon zest and season with salt and pepper to taste. Serve salmon with cauliflower,

sprinkling individual portions with scallions and sesame seeds.

Grilled Fish on Lemons

PREP TIME: 10 MINUTES / COOK TIME: 10 MINUTES/ SERVES 4

Ingredients

4 (4-ounce) fish fillets, such as tilapia, salmon, catfish, cod, or your favorite fish
Nonstick cooking spray
3 to 4 medium lemons
1 tablespoon extra-virgin olive oil
¼ teaspoon freshly ground black pepper
¼ teaspoon kosher or sea salt

Directions

1. **Preparing the Ingredients**

Using paper towels, pat the fillets dry and let stand at room temperature for 10 minutes. Meanwhile, coat the cold cooking grate of the grill with nonstick cooking spray, and preheat the grill to 400°F, or medium-high heat. Or preheat a grill pan over medium-high heat on the stove top. Cut one lemon in half and set half aside. Slice the remaining half of that lemon and the remaining lemons into ¼-inch-thick slices. (You should have about 12 to 16 lemon slices.) Into a small bowl, squeeze 1 tablespoon of juice out of the reserved lemon half. Add the oil to the bowl with the lemon juice, and mix well. Brush both sides of the fish with the oil mixture, and sprinkle evenly with pepper and salt. Carefully place the lemon slices on the grill (or the grill pan), arranging 3 to 4 slices together in the shape of a fish fillet, and repeat with the remaining slices.

2. **Cooking**

Place the fish fillets directly on top of the lemon slices, and grill with the lid closed. (If you're grilling on the stove top, cover with a large pot lid or aluminum foil.) Turn the fish halfway through the cooking time only if the fillets are more than half an inch thick. The fish is done and ready to serve when it just begins to separate into flakes (chunks) when pressed gently with a fork.

Salmon Cakes with Bell Pepper and Lemon Yogurt

PREP TIME: 15 MINUTES / COOK TIME: 15 MINUTES/SERVES 4

Ingredients

¼ cup whole-wheat bread crumbs
¼ cup mayonnaise
1 large egg, beaten
1 tablespoon chives, chopped
1 tablespoon fresh parsley, chopped
Zest of 1 lemon
¾ teaspoon kosher salt, divided
¼ teaspoon freshly ground black pepper
2 (5- to 6-ounce) cans no-salt boneless/skinless salmon, drained and finely flaked
½ bell pepper, diced small
2 tablespoons extra-virgin olive oil, divided

1 cup plain Greek yogurt
Juice of 1 lemon

Directions

1. **Preparing the Ingredients**
In a large bowl, combine the bread crumbs, mayonnaise, egg, chives, parsley, lemon zest, ½ teaspoon of the salt, and black pepper and mix well. Add the salmon and the bell pepper and stir gently until well combined. Shape the mixture into 8 patties.
2. **Cooking** Heat 1 tablespoon of the olive oil in a large skillet over medium-high heat. Cook half the cakes until the bottoms are golden brown, 4 to 5 minutes. Adjust the heat to medium if the bottoms start to burn. Flip the cakes and cook until golden brown, an additional 4 to 5 minutes. Repeat with the remaining 1 tablespoon olive oil and the rest of the cakes.
In a small bowl, combine the yogurt, lemon juice, and the remaining ¼ teaspoon salt and mix well. Serve with the salmon cakes.

Shrimp Mojo de Ajo

PREP TIME: 10 MINUTES / COOK TIME: 40 MINUTES/ SERVES 4

Ingredients
¼ cup extra-virgin olive oil
10 garlic cloves, minced
⅛ teaspoon cayenne pepper, plus more as needed
8 ounces mushrooms, quartered
1 pound medium shrimp, peeled, deveined, and tails removed
Juice of 1 lime
½ teaspoon sea salt
¼ cup chopped fresh cilantro leaves
2 cups cooked brown rice

Directions

1. **Preparing the Ingredients**. In a small saucepan over the lowest heat setting, bring the olive oil, garlic, and cayenne to a low simmer so bubbles just barely break the surface of the oil. Simmer for 30 minutes, stirring occasionally. Strain the garlic from the oil and set it aside.
2. **Cooking**. Add the olive oil to a large skillet over medium-high heat and heat it until it shimmers. Add the mushrooms. Cook for about 5 minutes, stirring once or twice, until browned. Add the shrimp, lime juice, and sea salt. Cook for about 4 minutes, stirring occasionally, until the shrimp are pink. Remove from the heat and stir in the cilantro and reserved garlic. Serve over the hot brown rice.

Easy Shrimp Paella

PREP TIME: 20 MINUTES / COOK TIME: 1 HOUR 5 MINUTES / SERVES 2

Ingredients
2 tablespoons olive oil
½ large onion, minced
1 garlic clove, minced
4 ounces chorizo sausage, removed from casing
1 cup diced tomato (about 1 medium tomato)
½ teaspoon sweet paprika
Generous pinch saffron
½ cup medium- or short-grain rice
½ cup dry white wine
1¼ cups low-sodium chicken stock
8 ounces large raw shrimp
1 cup frozen peas
¼ cup jarred roasted red peppers, cut into strips (about 1 whole pepper)
Salt

Directions

1. **Preparing the Ingredients**. Heat the olive oil in a large sauté pan over medium-high heat. Add the onion, garlic, and chorizo, and sauté for 10 minutes, or until the onion is wilted and the chorizo is cooked. Add the tomato, paprika, saffron, and rice, and stir for 3 minutes to toast the rice and spices. Add the wine and chicken stock and stir. Bring the mixture to a boil. Cover and reduce the heat to medium-low, and let the paella cook for 45 minutes, or until the rice is just about tender and most, but not all, of the liquid has been absorbed. Add the shrimp, peas, and roasted red peppers. Cover and cook for another 5 minutes. Season with salt.

Salmon with Garlicky Broccoli Rabe and White Beans (Instant Pot)

PREP TIME: 22 MINUTES / COOK TIME: 3 MINUTES/ SERVES 4

Ingredients
2 tablespoons extra-virgin olive oil, plus extra for drizzling
4 garlic cloves, sliced thin
½ cup chicken or vegetable broth
¼ teaspoon red pepper flakes
1 lemon, sliced ¼ inch thick, plus lemon wedges for serving
4 (6-ounce) skinless salmon fillets, 1½ inches thick
½ teaspoon table salt
¼ teaspoon pepper
1 pound broccoli rabe, trimmed and cut into 1-inch pieces
1 (15-ounce) can cannellini beans, rinsed

Directions

Preparing the Ingredients

1. Using highest sauté function, cook oil and garlic in Instant Pot until garlic is fragrant and light golden brown, about 3 minutes. Using slotted spoon, transfer garlic to paper towel–lined plate and season with salt to taste; set aside for serving. Turn off Instant Pot, then stir in broth and pepper flakes. Fold sheet of aluminum foil into 16 by 6-inch sling. Arrange lemon slices widthwise in 2 rows across center of sling. Sprinkle flesh side of salmon with salt and pepper, then arrange skinned side down on top of lemon slices. Using sling, lower salmon into Instant Pot; allow narrow edges of sling to rest along sides of insert. Lock lid in place and close pressure release valve. Select high pressure cook function and cook for 3 minutes.

2.	Turn off Instant Pot and quick-release pressure. Carefully remove lid, allowing steam to escape away from you. Using sling, transfer salmon to large plate. Tent with foil and let rest while preparing broccoli rabe mixture.

3.	Stir broccoli rabe and beans into cooking liquid, partially cover, and cook, using highest sauté function, until broccoli rabe is tender, about 5 minutes. Season with salt and pepper to taste. Gently lift and tilt salmon fillets with spatula to remove lemon slices. Serve salmon with broccoli rabe mixture and lemon wedges, sprinkling individual portions with garlic chips and drizzling with extra oil.

Weeknight Sheet Pan Fish Dinner

PREP TIME: 10 MINUTES / COOK TIME: 10 MINUTES/ SERVES 4

Ingredients
Nonstick cooking spray
2 tablespoons extra-virgin olive oil
1 tablespoon balsamic vinegar
4 (4-ounce) fish fillets, such as cod or tilapia (½ inch thick)
2½ cups green beans (about 12 ounces)
1 pint cherry or grape tomatoes (about 2 cups)

Directions

**1.	Preparing the Ingredients**
Preheat the oven to 400°F. Coat two large, rimmed baking sheets with nonstick cooking spray. In a small bowl, whisk together the oil and vinegar. Set aside.
Place two pieces of fish on each baking sheet.
In a large bowl, combine the beans and tomatoes.
Pour in the oil and vinegar, and toss gently to coat.
Pour half of the green bean mixture over the fish on one baking sheet, and the remaining half over the fish on the other.
Turn the fish over, and rub it in the oil mixture to coat.
Spread the vegetables evenly on the baking sheets so hot air can circulate around them.

**2.	Cooking**
Bake for 5 to 8 minutes, until the fish is just opaque and not translucent.
The fish is done and ready to serve when it just begins to separate into flakes (chunks) when pressed gently with a fork.

Halibut in Parchment with Zucchini, Shallots, and Herbs

PREP TIME: 15 MINUTES / COOK TIME: 15 MINUTES / SERVES 4

Ingredients
½ cup zucchini, diced small
1 shallot, minced
4 (5-ounce) halibut fillets (about 1 inch thick)
4 teaspoons extra-virgin olive oil
¼ teaspoon kosher salt
⅛ teaspoon freshly ground black pepper
1 lemon, sliced into ⅛-inch-thick rounds

8 sprigs of thyme

Directions

**1.	Preparing the Ingredients**
Preheat the oven to 450°F. Combine the zucchini and shallots in a medium bowl.
Cut 4 (15-by-24-inch) pieces of parchment paper. Fold each sheet in half horizontally. Draw a large half heart on one side of each folded sheet, with the fold along the center of the heart. Cut out the heart, open the parchment, and lay it flat.
Place a fillet near the center of each parchment heart. Drizzle 1 teaspoon olive oil on each fillet. Sprinkle with salt and pepper. Top each fillet with lemon slices and 2 sprigs of thyme. Sprinkle each fillet with one-quarter of the zucchini and shallot mixture. Fold the parchment over. Starting at the top, fold the edges of the parchment over, and continue all the way around to make a packet. Twist the end tightly to secure.

**2.	Cooking**
Arrange the 4 packets on a baking sheet. Bake for about 15 minutes. Place on plates; cut open. Serve immediately.

Pan-Seared Scallops with Sautéed Spinach

PREP TIME: 10 MINUTES / COOK TIME: 15 MINUTES/ SERVES 4

Ingredients
1 pound sea scallops
1 teaspoon sea salt, divided
½ teaspoon freshly ground black pepper, divided
2 tablespoons extra-virgin olive oil
6 cups fresh baby spinach
Juice of 1 orange
Pinch red pepper flakes

Directions

**1.	Preparing the Ingredients**
Season the scallops on both sides with ½ teaspoon of sea salt and ¼ teaspoon of pepper. In a large skillet over medium-high heat, heat the olive oil until it shimmers.

**2.	Cooking**
Add the scallops. Cook for 3 to 4 minutes per side without moving until browned. Remove the scallops from the skillet and set aside, tented with aluminum foil to keep warm.
Return the skillet to the heat and add the spinach, orange juice, red pepper flakes, remaining ½ teaspoon of salt, and remaining ¼ teaspoon of pepper.
Cook for 4 to 5 minutes, stirring, until the spinach wilts. Divide the spinach among 4 plates and top with the scallops. Serve immediately.

Salmon with Wild Rice and Orange Salad (Instant Pot)

PREP TIME: 38 MINUTES / COOK TIME: 38 MINUTES/ SERVES 4

Ingredients
1 cup wild rice, picked over and rinsed

3 tablespoons extra-virgin olive oil, divided
1½ teaspoon table salt, for cooking rice
2 oranges, plus ⅛ teaspoon grated orange zest
4 (6-ounce) skinless salmon fillets, 1½ inches thick
1 teaspoon ground dried Aleppo pepper
½ teaspoon table salt
1 small shallot, minced
1 tablespoon red wine vinegar
2 teaspoons Dijon mustard
1 teaspoon honey
2 carrots, peeled and shredded
¼ cup chopped fresh mint

Directions
Preparing the Ingredients
1.   Combine 6 cups water, rice, 1 tablespoon oil, and 1½ teaspoons salt in Instant Pot. Lock lid in place and close pressure release valve. Select high pressure cook function and cook for 15 minutes.
2.   Turn off Instant Pot and let pressure release naturally for 15 minutes. Quick-release any remaining pressure, then carefully remove lid, allowing steam to escape away from you. Drain rice and set aside to cool slightly. Wipe pot clean with paper towels. Add ½ cup water to now-empty Instant Pot. Fold sheet of aluminum foil into 16 by 6-inch sling. Slice 1 orange ¼ inch thick and shingle widthwise in 3 rows across center of sling. Sprinkle flesh side of salmon with Aleppo pepper and ½ teaspoon salt, then arrange skinned side down on top of orange slices. Using sling, lower salmon into Instant Pot; allow narrow edges of sling to rest along sides of insert.
3.   Lock lid in place and close pressure release valve. Select high pressure cook function and cook for 3 minutes. Meanwhile, cut away peel and pith from remaining 1 orange. Quarter orange, then slice crosswise into ¼-inch pieces.
Whisk remaining 2 tablespoons oil, shallot, vinegar, mustard, honey, and orange zest together in large bowl.
4.   Add rice, orange pieces, carrots, and mint, and gently toss to combine. Season with salt and pepper to taste.
5.   Turn off Instant Pot and quick-release pressure. Carefully remove lid, allowing steam to escape away from you. Using sling, transfer salmon to large plate. Gently lift and tilt fillets with spatula to remove orange slices.
Serve salmon with salad.

Crispy Polenta Fish Sticks

PREP TIME: 15 MINUTES / COOK TIME: 10 MINUTES/ SERVES 4
Ingredients
2 large eggs, lightly beaten 1 tablespoon 2% milk
1 pound skinned fish fillets (cod, tilapia, or other white fish) about ½ inch thick, sliced into 20 (1-inch-wide) strips
½ cup yellow cornmeal

½ cup whole-wheat panko bread crumbs or whole-wheat bread crumbs
¼ teaspoon smoked paprika
¼ teaspoon kosher or sea salt
¼ teaspoon freshly ground black pepper
Nonstick cooking spray

Directions
1.   Preparing the Ingredients
Place a large, rimmed baking sheet in the oven. Preheat the oven to 400°F with the pan inside. In a large bowl, mix the eggs and milk. Using a fork, add the fish strips to the egg mixture and stir gently to coat. Put the cornmeal, bread crumbs, smoked paprika, salt, and pepper in a quart-size zip-top plastic bag.
Using a fork or tongs, transfer the fish to the bag, letting the excess egg wash drip off into the bowl before transferring. Seal the bag and shake gently to completely coat each fish stick.
With oven mitts, carefully remove the hot baking sheet from the oven and spray it with nonstick cooking spray. Using a fork or tongs, remove the fish sticks from the bag and arrange them on the hot baking sheet, with space between them so the hot air can circulate and crisp them up.
2.   Cooking
Bake for 5 to 8 minutes, until gentle pressure with a fork causes the fish to flake, and serve.

Flounder with Tomatoes and Basil

PREP TIME: 10 MINUTES / COOK TIME: 20 MINUTES/ SERVES 4
Ingredients
1 pound cherry tomatoes
4 garlic cloves, sliced
2 tablespoons extra-virgin olive oil
2 tablespoons lemon juice
2 tablespoons basil, cut into ribbons
½ teaspoon kosher salt
¼ teaspoon freshly ground black pepper
4 (5- to 6-ounce) flounder fillets

Directions
1.   Preparing the Ingredients
Preheat the oven to 425°F. In a baking dish, combine the tomatoes, garlic, olive oil, lemon juice, basil, salt, and black pepper; mix well.
2.   **Cooking**. Bake for 5 minutes. Remove the baking dish from the oven and arrange the flounder on top of the tomato mixture. Bake until the fish is opaque and begins to flake, about 10 to 15 minutes, depending on thickness.
Halibut or sole can be used in this dish in place of flounder.

Pan-Roasted Salmon with Gremolata

PREP TIME: 10 MINUTES / COOK TIME: 10 MINUTES/ SERVES 6
Ingredients
1½ pounds skin-on salmon fillet, cut into 4 pieces
1 teaspoon sea salt, divided

¼ teaspoon freshly ground black pepper
3 tablespoons extra-virgin olive oil
1 bunch fresh Italian parsley leaves, finely chopped
1 garlic clove, minced
Zest of 1 lemon, finely grated

Directions

1.   Preparing the Ingredients
Preheat the oven to 350°F. Season the salmon with ½ teaspoon of salt and the pepper.
In a large, ovenproof skillet over medium-high heat, heat the olive oil until it shimmers.
Add the salmon to the skillet, skin-side down.

2.   Cooking
Cook for about 5 minutes, gently pressing on the salmon with a spatula, until the skin crisps. Transfer the pan to the oven and cook the salmon for 3 to 4 minutes more until it is opaque.
In a small bowl, stir together the parsley, garlic, lemon zest, and remaining ½ teaspoon of sea salt. Sprinkle the mixture over the salmon and serve.

Seared Scallops with White Bean Purée

PREP TIME: 15 MINUTES / COOK TIME: 15 MINUTES / SERVES 2

Ingredients
4 tablespoons olive oil, divided
2 garlic cloves
2 teaspoons minced fresh rosemary
1 (15-ounce) can white cannellini beans, drained and rinsed
½ cup low-sodium chicken stock
Salt
Freshly ground black pepper
10 ounces sea scallops (about 6)

Directions

Preparing the Ingredients
1.   To make the bean purée, heat 2 tablespoons of olive oil in a saucepan over medium-high heat. Add the garlic and sauté for 30 seconds, or just until it's fragrant. Don't let it burn. Add the rosemary and remove the pan from the heat.
Add the white beans and chicken stock to the pan, return it to the heat, and stir. Bring the beans to a boil. Reduce the heat to low and simmer for 5 minutes. Transfer the beans to a blender and purée them for 30 seconds, or until they're smooth. Taste and season with salt and pepper. Let them sit in the blender with the lid on to keep them warm while you prepare the scallops. Pat the scallops dry with a paper towel and season them with salt and pepper.
2.   Heat the remaining 2 tablespoons of olive oil in a large sauté pan. When the oil is shimmering, add the scallops, flat-side down. Cook the scallops for 2 minutes, or until they're golden on the bottom. Flip them over and cook for another 1 to 2 minutes, or until opaque and slightly firm. To serve, divide the bean purée between two plates and top with the scallops.

Grilled Mahi-Mahi with Artichoke Caponata

PREP TIME: 25 MINUTES / COOK TIME: 30 MINUTES / SERVES 4

Ingredients
2 tablespoons extra-virgin olive oil
2 celery stalks, diced
1 onion, diced
2 garlic cloves, minced
½ cup cherry tomatoes, chopped
¼ cup white wine
2 tablespoons white wine vinegar
1 (14-ounce) can artichoke hearts, drained and chopped
¼ cup green olives, pitted and chopped
1 tablespoon capers, chopped
¼ teaspoon red pepper flakes
2 tablespoons fresh basil, chopped
4 (5- to 6-ounces each) skinless mahi-mahi fillets
½ teaspoon kosher salt
¼ teaspoon freshly ground black pepper
Olive oil cooking spray

Directions

Preparing the Ingredients
1.   Heat the olive oil in a large skillet or sauté pan over medium heat. Add the celery and onion, and sauté 4 to 5 minutes. Add the garlic and sauté 30 seconds. Add the tomatoes and cook 2 to 3 minutes. Add the wine and vinegar to deglaze the pan, increasing the heat to medium-high and scraping up any brown bits on the bottom of the pan.
2.   Add the artichokes, olives, capers, and red pepper flakes and simmer, reducing the liquid by half, about 10 minutes. Mix in the basil.
3.   Season the mahi-mahi with the salt and pepper. Heat a grill skillet or grill pan over medium-high heat and coat with olive oil cooking spray. Add the fish and cook 4 to 5 minutes per side. Serve topped with the artichoke caponata.

Salmon Burgers

PREP TIME: 10 MINUTES / COOK TIME: 10 MINUTES/ SERVES 6

Ingredients
16 ounces canned salmon, drained
6 scallions, white and green parts, finely chopped
¼ cup whole-wheat bread crumbs
2 eggs, beaten
2 tablespoons chopped fresh Italian parsley leaves
1 tablespoon dried Italian seasoning
Zest of 1 lemon
2 tablespoons extra-virgin olive oil
¼ cup unsweetened nonfat plain Greek yogurt
1 tablespoon chopped fresh dill
1 tablespoon capers, rinsed and chopped
¼ teaspoon sea salt
6 whole-wheat hamburger buns

Directions

1. **Preparing the Ingredients**. In a medium bowl, mix together the salmon, scallions, bread crumbs, eggs, parsley, Italian seasoning, and lemon zest. Form the mixture into 6 patties about ½-inch thick. In a large nonstick skillet over medium-high heat, heat the olive oil until it shimmers.

2. **Cooking.** Add the salmon patties. Cook for about 4 minutes per side until browned.

While the salmon cooks, in a small bowl, whisk the yogurt, dill, capers, and sea salt. Spread the sauce on the buns. Top with the patties and serve.

Lemon Pesto Salmon

PREP TIME: 5 MINUTES / COOK TIME: 10 MINUTES/ SERVES 2
Ingredients
10 ounces salmon fillet (1 large piece or 2 smaller ones)
Salt
Freshly ground black pepper
2 tablespoons prepared pesto sauce
1 large fresh lemon, sliced
Directions
1. **Preparing the Ingredients**
Oil the grill grate and heat the grill to medium-high heat. Alternatively, you can roast the salmon in a 350°F oven. Prepare the salmon by seasoning with salt and freshly ground black pepper, and then spread the pesto sauce on top. Make a bed of fresh lemon slices about the same size as your fillet on the hot grill (or on a baking sheet if roasting), and rest the salmon on top of the lemon slices. Place any additional lemon slices on top of the salmon.

2. **Cooking.** Grill the salmon for 6 to 10 minutes, or until it's opaque and flakes apart easily. If roasting, it will take about 20 minutes. There is no need to flip the fish over. Salmon should be cooked to an internal temperature of 145°F. Keep in mind that a thicker piece of fish will take longer to cook. Purchasing pesto, check the ingredients to make sure it's made with olive oil and not corn or soybean oil. Also check to see if it contains salt—if so, you'll need less salt to season your salmon.

Hake in Saffron Broth (Instant Pot)

PREP TIME: 30 MINUTES / COOK TIME: 30 MINUTES/ SERVES 4
Ingredients
2 tablespoons extra-virgin olive oil, divided, plus extra for drizzling
1 onion, chopped
4 ounces Spanish-style chorizo sausage, sliced ¼ inch thick
4 garlic cloves, minced
1 (8-ounce) bottle clam juice
¾ cup water
½ cup dry white wine
8 ounces small red potatoes, unpeeled, quartered
¼ teaspoon saffron threads, crumbled
1 bay leaf

4 (6-ounce) skinless hake fillets, 1½ inches thick
½ teaspoon table salt
¼ teaspoon pepper
2 tablespoons minced fresh parsley
Directions
1. Using highest sauté function, heat 1 tablespoon oil in Instant Pot until shimmering. Add onion and chorizo and cook until onion is softened and lightly browned, 5 to 7 minutes. Stir in garlic and cook until fragrant, about 30 seconds. Stir in clam juice, water, and wine, scraping up any browned bits. Turn off Instant Pot, then stir in potatoes, saffron, and bay leaf.

2. Fold sheet of aluminum foil into 16 by 6-inch sling. Brush hake with remaining 1 tablespoon oil and sprinkle with salt and pepper. Arrange hake skinned side down in center of sling. Using sling, lower hake into Instant Pot on top of potato mixture; allow narrow edges of sling to rest along sides of insert. Lock lid in place and close pressure release valve. Select high pressure cook function and cook for 3 minutes.

3. Turn off Instant Pot and quick-release pressure. Carefully remove lid, allowing steam to escape away from you. Using sling, transfer hake to large plate. Tent with aluminum foil and let rest while finishing potato mixture.

4. Discard bay leaf. Stir parsley into potato mixture and season with salt to taste. Serve cod with potato mixture and broth, drizzling individual portions with extra oil.

Tuscan Tuna and Zucchini Burgers

PREP TIME: 10 MINUTES / COOK TIME: 10 MINUTES/ SERVES 4
Ingredients
3 slices whole-wheat sandwich bread, toasted
2 (5-ounce) cans tuna in olive oil, drained
1 cup shredded zucchini (about ¾ small zucchini)
1 large egg, lightly beaten
¼ cup diced red bell pepper (about ¼ pepper)
1 tablespoon dried oregano
1 teaspoon lemon zest
¼ teaspoon freshly ground black pepper
¼ teaspoon kosher or sea salt
1 tablespoon extra-virgin olive oil
Salad greens or 4 whole-wheat rolls, for serving (optional)
Directions
1. **Preparing the Ingredients**
Crumble the toast into bread crumbs using your fingers (or use a knife to cut into ¼-inch cubes) until you have 1 cup of loosely packed crumbs. Pour the crumbs into a large bowl. Add the tuna, zucchini, egg, bell pepper, oregano, lemon zest, black pepper, and salt. Mix well with a fork. With your hands, form the mixture into four (½-cup-size) patties.

Place on a plate, and press each patty flat to about ¾-inch thick.

2. **Cooking**

In a large skillet over medium-high heat, heat the oil until it's very hot, about 2 minutes. Add the patties to the hot oil, then turn the heat down to medium. Cook the patties for 5 minutes, flip with a spatula, and cook for an additional 5 minutes. Enjoy as is or serve on salad greens or whole-wheat rolls.

Cod and Cauliflower Chowder

PREP TIME: 15 MINUTES / COOK TIME: 40 MINUTES / SERVES 4

Ingredients

2 tablespoons extra-virgin olive oil
1 leek, white and light green parts only, cut in half lengthwise and sliced thinly
4 garlic cloves, sliced
1 medium head cauliflower, coarsely chopped
1 teaspoon kosher salt
¼ teaspoon freshly ground black pepper
2 pints cherry tomatoes
2 cups no-salt-added vegetable stock
¼ cup green olives, pitted and chopped
1 to 1½ pounds cod
¼ cup fresh parsley, minced

Directions

Preparing the Ingredients

1.   Heat the olive oil in a Dutch oven or large pot over medium heat. Add the leek and sauté until lightly golden brown, about 5 minutes. Add the garlic and sauté for 30 seconds. Add the cauliflower, salt, and black pepper and sauté 2 to 3 minutes.

2.   Add the tomatoes and vegetable stock, increase the heat to high and bring to a boil, then turn the heat to low and simmer for 10 minutes.

3.   Add the olives and mix together. Add the fish, cover, and simmer 20 minutes, or until fish is opaque and flakes easily. Gently mix in the parsley.

Crab Cakes with Shaved Fennel Salad

PREP TIME: 20 MINUTES / COOK TIME: 10 MINUTES / SERVES 6

Ingredients

¾ cup cooked baby shrimp
3 tablespoons heavy (whipping) cream
1 teaspoon sea salt, divided
¼ teaspoon freshly ground black pepper, divided
1½ pounds lump crabmeat
6 scallions, white and green parts, thinly sliced
¼ cup extra-virgin olive oil, divided
3 fennel bulbs, cored and very thinly sliced
2 tablespoons chopped fennel fronds
¼ cup freshly squeezed lemon juice
½ teaspoon Dijon mustard
1 garlic clove, minced

Directions

1.   **Preparing the Ingredients**

In a blender or food processor, blend the shrimp, heavy cream, ½ teaspoon of sea salt, and ⅛ teaspoon of pepper until smooth. In a large bowl, stir together the crabmeat and scallions. Fold in the shrimp

mousse until well mixed. Form the mixture into 8 patties. Refrigerate for 10 minutes.

2.   **Cooking**

In a large, nonstick skillet over medium-high heat, heat 2 tablespoons of olive oil until it shimmers. Add the crab cakes.

Cook for about 4 minutes per side until browned on both sides.

In a large bowl, combine the fennel and fennel fronds. In a small bowl, whisk the remaining 2 tablespoons of olive oil with the lemon juice, mustard, garlic, and remaining ½ teaspoon of sea salt, and ⅛ teaspoon of pepper. Toss the dressing with the fennel and serve with the crab cakes.

If you have a mandoline, save some time by setting it to ⅛ inch and shaving the fennel. You can also use the shaving part of a box grater, or use a slicer in a food processor.

Shrimp with Arugula Pesto and Zucchini Noodles

PREP TIME: 20 MINUTES / COOK TIME: 5 MINUTES/ SERVES 2

Ingredients

3 cups lightly packed arugula
½ cup lightly packed basil leaves
3 medium garlic cloves
¼ cup walnuts
3 tablespoons olive oil
2 tablespoons grated Parmesan cheese
1 tablespoon freshly squeezed lemon juice
Salt
Freshly ground black pepper
1 (10-ounce) package zucchini noodles
8 ounces cooked, shelled shrimp
2 Roma tomatoes, diced

Directions

1.   **Preparing the Ingredients**

Combine the arugula, basil, garlic, walnuts, olive oil, Parmesan cheese, and lemon juice in a food processor fitted with the chopping blade. Process until smooth, scraping down the sides as needed. Season with salt and pepper.

2.   **Cooking**

Heat a sauté pan over medium heat. Add the pesto, zucchini noodles, and shrimp. Toss to combine the sauce over the noodles and shrimp, and cook until warmed through. Don't overcook or the zucchini will become limp.

Taste and add additional salt and pepper if needed. Top with the diced tomatoes.

To make this dairy-free, substitute nutritional yeast for the Parmesan cheese.

If you don't have a food processor, use a blender to make the pesto. Just make sure you scrape down the sides often.

Braised Striped Bass with Zucchini and Tomatoes (Instant Pot)

PREP TIME: 30 MINUTES / COOK TIME: 30 MINUTES/ SERVES 4

Ingredients

2 tablespoons extra-virgin olive oil, divided, plus extra for drizzling
3 zucchini (8 ounces each), halved lengthwise and sliced ¼ inch thick
1 onion, chopped
¾ teaspoon table salt, divided
3 garlic cloves, minced
1 teaspoon minced fresh oregano or ¼ teaspoon dried
¼ teaspoon red pepper flakes
1 (28-ounce) can whole peeled tomatoes, drained with juice reserved, halved
1½ pounds skinless striped bass, 1½ inches thick, cut into 2-inch pieces
¼ teaspoon pepper
2 tablespoons chopped pitted kalamata olives
2 tablespoons shredded fresh mint

Directions

1.   Using highest sauté function, heat 1 tablespoon oil in Instant Pot for 5 minutes (or until just smoking). Add zucchini and cook until tender, about 5 minutes; transfer to bowl and set aside. Add remaining 1 tablespoon oil, onion, and ¼ teaspoon salt to now-empty pot and cook, using highest sauté function, until onion is softened, about 5 minutes. Stir in garlic, oregano, and pepper flakes and cook until fragrant, about 30 seconds. Stir in tomatoes and reserved juice.

2.   Sprinkle bass with remaining ½ teaspoon salt and pepper. Nestle bass into tomato mixture and spoon some of cooking liquid on top of pieces. Lock lid in place and close pressure release valve. Select high pressure cook function and set cook time for 0 minutes. Once Instant Pot has reached pressure, immediately turn off pot and quick-release pressure. Carefully remove lid, allowing steam to escape away from you.

3.   Transfer bass to plate, tent with aluminum foil, and let rest while finishing vegetables. Stir zucchini into pot and let sit until heated through, about 5 minutes. Stir in olives and season with salt and pepper to taste. Serve bass with vegetables, sprinkling individual portions with mint and drizzling with extra oil.

Sardine Bruschetta with Fennel and Lemon Crema

PREP TIME: 15 MINUTES / COOK TIME: 0 MINUTES/ SERVES 4

Ingredients

⅓ cup plain Greek yogurt
2 tablespoons mayonnaise
2 tablespoons lemon juice, divided
2 teaspoons lemon zest
¾ teaspoon kosher salt, divided
1 fennel bulb, cored and thinly sliced
¼ cup fresh parsley, chopped, plus more for garnish
¼ cup fresh mint, chopped, plus more for garnish
2 teaspoons extra-virgin olive oil
⅛ teaspoon freshly ground black pepper
8 slices multigrain bread, toasted
2 (4.4-ounce) cans smoked sardines

Directions

1.   **Preparing the Ingredients**

In a small bowl, combine the yogurt, mayonnaise, 1 tablespoon of the lemon juice, the lemon zest, and ¼ teaspoon of the salt. In a separate small bowl, combine the remaining ½ teaspoon salt, the remaining 1 tablespoon lemon juice, the fennel, parsley, mint, olive oil, and black pepper.

Spoon 1 tablespoon of the yogurt mixture on each piece of toast.

Divide the fennel mixture evenly on top of the yogurt mixture.

Divide the sardines among the toasts, placing them on top of the fennel mixture.

Garnish with more herbs, if desired. Other smoked fish, including smoked trout or smoked salmon, would also work well in this dish.

Swordfish Kebabs

PREP TIME: 20 MINUTES / COOK TIME: 10 MINUTES/ SERVES 6

Ingredients

3 tablespoons extra-virgin olive oil, plus more for the grill
Juice of 2 oranges
1 tablespoon Dijon mustard
2 teaspoons dried tarragon
½ teaspoon sea salt
⅛ teaspoon freshly ground black pepper
2 pounds swordfish, cut into 1½-inch pieces
2 red bell peppers, cut into pieces

Directions

1.   **Preparing the Ingredients**

In a medium bowl, whisk the olive oil, orange juice, mustard, tarragon, sea salt, and pepper.

Add the swordfish and toss to coat. Let sit for 10 minutes.

2.   **Cooking**

Heat a grill or grill pan to medium-high heat and brush it with oil.

Thread the swordfish and red bell peppers onto 6 wooden skewers.

Cook for 6 to 8 minutes, turning, until the fish is opaque. Serve these kebabs with Rice and Spinach. Soak your wooden skewers in water before threading the food on them to prevent burning on the grill.

Salmon Cakes with Tzatziki Sauce

PREP TIME: 20 MINUTES / COOK TIME: 10 MINUTES/ SERVES 6

Ingredients

½ cup plain Greek yogurt
1 teaspoon dried dill
¼ cup minced cucumber

Salt
Freshly ground black pepper
6 ounces cooked salmon (or 8 ounces raw)
3 tablespoons olive oil, divided
¼ cup minced celery
¼ cup minced onion
½ teaspoon dried dill
1 tablespoon fresh minced parsley
Salt
Freshly ground black pepper
1 egg, beaten
½ cup unseasoned bread crumbs

Directions

1.   Preparing the Ingredients
Combine the yogurt, dill, and cucumber in a small bowl. Season with salt and pepper and set aside. Remove any skin from the salmon. Place the salmon in a medium bowl and break it into small flakes with a fork. Set it aside.

2.   Cooking. Heat 1 tablespoon of olive oil in a nonstick skillet over medium-high heat. Add the celery and onion and sauté for 5 minutes.

Add the celery and onion to the salmon and stir to combine. Add the dill and parsley, and season with salt and pepper.

Add the beaten egg and bread crumbs and stir until mixed thoroughly.

Wipe the skillet clean and add the remaining 2 tablespoons of oil. Heat the pan over medium-high heat.

Form the salmon mixture into 4 patties, and place them two at a time into the hot pan.

Cook for 3 minutes per side, or until they're golden brown. Carefully flip them over with a spatula and cook for another 3 minutes on the second side.

Repeat with the remaining salmon cakes and serve topped with the tzatziki sauce.

If you are starting with raw salmon, roast a salmon fillet in a 350°F oven for 20 minutes, or until fish flakes easily. Then, proceed with the rest of the recipe as written.

If you prefer, you can make these with canned salmon instead of fresh.

Halibut with Carrots, White Beans, and Chermoula (Instant Pot)

PREP TIME: 22 MINUTES / COOK TIME: 2 MINUTES/ SERVES 4

Ingredients
1 shallot, sliced thin
1 tablespoon extra-virgin olive oil
2 teaspoons lemon juice
1 pound carrots, peeled
1 (15-ounce) can navy beans, rinsed
½ cup chicken or vegetable broth
4 (6-ounce) skinless halibut fillets, 1½ inches thick
3 tablespoons Chermoula (this page), divided
¼ teaspoon table salt
1 cup fresh parsley or cilantro leaves
2 tablespoons sliced almonds, toasted

Directions

1.   Combine shallot, oil, and lemon juice in medium bowl; set aside. Cut carrots into 2-inch lengths. Leave thin pieces whole, halve medium pieces lengthwise, and quarter thick pieces lengthwise. Combine carrots, beans, and broth in Instant Pot.

2.   Fold sheet of aluminum foil into 16 by 6-inch sling. Brush halibut with 1 tablespoon Chermoula and sprinkle with salt. Arrange halibut skinned side down in center of sling. Using sling, lower halibut into Instant Pot on top of carrot mixture; allow narrow edges of sling to rest along sides of insert.

3.   Lock lid in place and close pressure release valve. Select high pressure cook function and set cook time for 0 minutes. Once Instant Pot has reached pressure, immediately turn off pot and quick-release pressure. Carefully remove lid, allowing steam to escape away from you.

4.   Using sling, transfer halibut to large plate. Tent with foil and let rest while finishing carrot mixture. Stir remaining 2 tablespoons Chermoula into carrot mixture and season with salt and pepper to taste. Add parsley and almonds to bowl with shallot mixture and gently toss to combine. Season with salt and pepper to taste. Serve halibut with carrot mixture, topped with parsley salad.

Mediterranean Cod Stew

PREP TIME: 10 MINUTES / COOK TIME: 20 MINUTES/ SERVES 6

Ingredients
2 tablespoons extra-virgin olive oil
2 cups chopped onion (about 1 medium onion)
2 garlic cloves, minced (about 1 teaspoon)
¾ teaspoon smoked paprika
1 (14.5-ounce) can diced tomatoes, undrained
1 (12-ounce) jar roasted red peppers, drained and chopped
1 cup sliced olives, green or black
⅓ cup dry red wine
¼ teaspoon freshly ground black pepper
¼ teaspoon kosher or sea salt
1½ pounds cod fillets, cut into 1-inch pieces
3 cups sliced mushrooms (about 8 ounces)

Directions

Preparing the Ingredients

1.   In a large stockpot over medium heat, heat the oil. Add the onion and cook for 4 minutes, stirring occasionally. Add the garlic and smoked paprika and cook for 1 minute, stirring often.

2.   Mix in the tomatoes with their juices, roasted peppers, olives, wine, pepper, and salt, and turn the heat up to medium-high. Bring to a boil. Add the cod and mushrooms, and reduce the heat to medium.

3.   Cover and cook for about 10 minutes, stirring a few times, until the cod is cooked through and flakes easily, and serve.

Chopped Tuna Salad

PREP TIME: 15 MINUTES / COOK TIME: 0 MINUTES/ SERVES 4

Ingredients

2 tablespoons extra-virgin olive oil
2 tablespoons lemon juice
2 teaspoons Dijon mustard
½ teaspoon kosher salt
¼ teaspoon freshly ground black pepper
12 olives, pitted and chopped
½ cup celery, diced
½ cup red onion, diced
½ cup red bell pepper, diced
½ cup fresh parsley, chopped
2 (6-ounce) cans no-salt-added tuna packed in water, drained
6 cups baby spinach

Directions
1.   Preparing the Ingredients
In a medium bowl, whisk together the olive oil, lemon juice, mustard, salt, and black pepper. Add in the olives, celery, onion, bell pepper, and parsley and mix well. Add the tuna and gently incorporate. Divide the spinach evenly among 4 plates or bowls. Spoon the tuna salad evenly on top of the spinach. Canned salmon can be used in place of canned tuna in this dish. Look for skinless, boneless salmon for the best results.

Cioppino

PREP TIME: 10 MINUTES / COOK TIME: 15 MINUTES/ SERVES 8
Ingredients
2 tablespoons extra-virgin olive oil
1 onion, chopped
1 fennel bulb, chopped
6 garlic cloves, minced
½ cup dry white wine
2 (32-ounce) cans tomato sauce
2 cups unsalted chicken broth
1 pound shrimp, peeled, deveined, and tails removed
1 pound cod, cut into bite-size pieces
1 pound salmon, skin removed, cut into bite-size pieces
2 tablespoons Italian seasoning
½ teaspoon sea salt
⅛ teaspoon red pepper flakes
⅛ teaspoon freshly ground black pepper
¼ cup chopped fresh basil leaves

Directions
Preparing the Ingredients
1.   In a large pot over medium-high heat, heat the olive oil until it shimmers.
Add the onion and fennel. Cook for about 5 minutes, stirring occasionally, until the vegetables are soft.
Add the garlic and cook for 30 seconds, stirring constantly.
2.   Stir in the wine and cook for 1 minute, stirring constantly.
Add the tomato sauce, broth, shrimp, cod, salmon, Italian seasoning, sea salt, red pepper flakes, and pepper. Bring to a simmer and reduce the heat to medium-low. Cook for about 5 minutes more, stirring occasionally, until the fish and shrimp are opaque.
Remove from heat and stir in the basil before serving.

Swordfish with Peppers and Potatoes (Instant Pot)

PREP TIME: 30 MINUTES / COOK TIME: 2 MINUTES/ SERVES 4
Ingredients
2 tablespoons extra-virgin olive oil
2 red bell peppers, stemmed, seeded, and cut into ½-inch-wide strips
2 green bell peppers, stemmed, seeded, and cut into ½-inch-wide strips
1 onion, halved and sliced thin
1 teaspoon table salt, divided
4 garlic cloves, minced
1 tablespoon tomato paste
1 teaspoon ground dried Espelette pepper, divided
1 (14.5-ounce) can whole peeled tomatoes, drained with ¼ cup juice reserved, chopped coarse
1 pound Yukon Gold potatoes, peeled, cut into 1-inch pieces
4 (6-ounce) skinless swordfish steaks, 1½ inches thick
¼ cup Salsa Verde

Directions
1.   Using highest sauté function, heat oil in Instant Pot until shimmering. Add bell peppers, onion, and ½ teaspoon salt and cook until vegetables are softened, about 5 minutes. Stir in garlic, tomato paste, and ½ teaspoon Espelette pepper and cook until fragrant, about 30 seconds.
Stir in tomatoes and reserved juice, scraping up any browned bits, then stir in potatoes. Sprinkle swordfish with remaining ½ teaspoon salt and remaining ½ teaspoon Espelette pepper. Nestle swordfish into vegetable mixture and spoon some of cooking liquid on top of steaks.
2.   Lock lid in place and close pressure release valve. Select high pressure cook function and set cook time for 0 minutes. Once Instant Pot has reached pressure, immediately turn off pot and quick-release pressure. Carefully remove lid, allowing steam to escape away from you.
3.   Using spatula, transfer swordfish to serving dish. Tent with aluminum foil and let rest while finishing vegetable mixture. Using highest sauté function, cook vegetable mixture until liquid has thickened slightly, about 2 minutes. Serve swordfish with vegetable mixture, drizzling individual portions with Salsa Verde.

Steamed Mussels in White Wine Sauce

PREP TIME: 5 MINUTES / COOK TIME: 10 MINUTES/ SERVES 2
Ingredients
2 pounds small mussels
1 tablespoon extra-virgin olive oil
1 cup thinly sliced red onion (about ½ medium onion)
3 garlic cloves, sliced (about 1½ teaspoons)
1 cup dry white wine
2 (¼-inch-thick) lemon slices
¼ teaspoon freshly ground black pepper
¼ teaspoon kosher or sea salt
Fresh lemon wedges, for serving (optional)

Directions
1.   Preparing the Ingredients
In a large colander in the sink, run cold water over the mussels (but don't let the mussels sit in standing

water). All the shells should be closed tight; discard any shells that are a little bit open or any shells that are cracked. Leave the mussels in the colander until you're ready to use them.

2.   Cooking

In a large skillet over medium-high heat, heat the oil. Add the onion and cook for 4 minutes, stirring occasionally. Add the garlic and cook for 1 minute, stirring constantly. Add the wine, lemon slices, pepper, and salt, and bring to a simmer. Cook for 2 minutes. Add the mussels and cover. Cook for 3 minutes, or until the mussels open their shells. Gently shake the pan two or three times while they are cooking.

All the shells should now be wide open. Using a slotted spoon, discard any mussels that are still closed. Spoon the opened mussels into a shallow serving bowl, and pour the broth over the top. Serve with additional fresh lemon slices, if desired.

Monkfish with Sautéed Leeks, Fennel, and Tomatoes

PREP TIME: 20 MINUTES / COOK TIME: 35 MINUTES/ SERVES 4

Ingredients

1 to 1½ pounds monkfish
3 tablespoons lemon juice, divided
1 teaspoon kosher salt, divided
⅛ teaspoon freshly ground black pepper
2 tablespoons extra-virgin olive oil
1 leek, white and light green parts only, sliced in half lengthwise and thinly sliced
½ onion, julienned
3 garlic cloves, minced
2 bulbs fennel, cored and thinly sliced, plus ¼ cup fronds for garnish
1 (14.5-ounce) can no-salt-added diced tomatoes
2 tablespoons fresh parsley, chopped
2 tablespoons fresh oregano, chopped
¼ teaspoon red pepper flakes

Directions

1.   Place the fish in a medium baking dish and add 2 tablespoons of the lemon juice, ¼ teaspoon of the salt, and the black pepper. Place in the refrigerator.

2.   Heat the olive oil in a large skillet or sauté pan over medium heat. Add the leek and onion and sauté until translucent, about 3 minutes. Add the garlic and sauté for 30 seconds. Add the fennel and sauté 4 to 5 minutes. Add the tomatoes and simmer for 2 to 3 minutes.

3.   Stir in the parsley, oregano, red pepper flakes, the remaining ¾ teaspoon salt, and the remaining 1 tablespoon lemon juice. Place the fish on top of the leek mixture, cover, and simmer for 20 to 25 minutes, turning over halfway through, until the fish is opaque and pulls apart easily. Garnish with the fennel fronds.

Switch the monkfish for sea bass, snapper, mahi-mahi, or halibut.

Halibut en Papillote with Capers, Onions, Olives, and Tomatoes

PREP TIME: 10 MINUTES / COOK TIME: 8 MINUTES / SERVES 4

Ingredients

4 (6-ounce) halibut fillets
2 tablespoons extra-virgin olive oil
½ teaspoon sea salt
¼ teaspoon freshly ground black pepper
⅛ teaspoon crushed red pepper flakes
2 garlic cloves, thinly sliced
1 cup grape tomatoes, halved
¼ cup chopped onion
2 tablespoons capers, drained
8 Kalamata olives, pitted and quartered
2 tablespoons plus 2 teaspoons dry white wine
8 fresh thyme sprigs

Directions

1.   **Preparing the Ingredients**

Cut 4 (15-inch) squares of parchment paper or aluminum foil. Set aside. Preheat the oven to 450°F. Brush the halibut with the olive oil and sprinkle with the sea salt, pepper, and red pepper flakes. Place each fillet on a parchment square.

2.   **Cooking.** Layer the fillets with the garlic, tomatoes, onion, capers, and olives. Fold into packets, leaving the tops open.

Add 2 teaspoons white wine to each packet along with a thyme sprig. Seal the packets and place them on a rimmed baking sheet. Bake for about 8 minutes until the fish is opaque. Serve immediately.

Roasted Branzino with Lemon and Herbs

PREP TIME: 10 MINUTES / COOK TIME: 20 MINUTES / SERVES 2

Ingredients

1 to 1½ pounds branzino, scaled and gutted
Salt
Freshly ground black pepper
1 tablespoon olive oil
1 lemon, sliced
3 garlic cloves, minced
¼ cup chopped fresh herbs (any mixture of oregano, thyme, parsley, and rosemary)

Directions

1.   **Preparing the Ingredients**

Preheat the oven to 425°F and set the rack to the middle position.

Lay the cleaned fish in a baking dish and make 4 to 5 slits in it, about 1½ inches apart.

Season the inside of the branzino with salt and pepper and drizzle with olive oil.

Fill the cavity of the fish with lemon slices. Sprinkle the chopped garlic and herbs over the lemon and close the fish.

2.   **Cooking**

Roast the fish for 15 to 20 minutes, or until the flesh is opaque and it flakes apart easily.

Before eating, open the fish, remove the lemon slices, and carefully pull out the bone.

POULTRY MAINS

Chicken Cutlets with Greek Salsa

PREP TIME: 15 MINUTES / COOK TIME: 30 MINUTES TO REST/ SERVES 2

Ingredients

2 tablespoons olive oil, divided
¼ teaspoon salt, plus additional to taste
Zest of ½ lemon
Juice of ½ lemon
8 ounces chicken cutlets, or chicken breast sliced through the middle to make 2 thin pieces
1 cup cherry or grape tomatoes, halved or quartered (about 4 ounces)
½ cup minced red onion (about ⅓ medium onion)
1 medium cucumber, peeled, seeded and diced (about 1 cup)
5 to 10 pitted Greek olives, minced (more or less depending on size and your taste)
1 tablespoon minced fresh parsley
1 tablespoon minced fresh oregano
1 tablespoon minced fresh mint
1 ounce crumbled feta cheese
1 tablespoon red wine vinegar

Directions

1. **Preparing the Ingredients**
In a medium bowl, combine 1 tablespoon of olive oil, the salt, lemon zest, and lemon juice. Add the chicken and let it marinate while you make the salsa.
In a small bowl, combine the tomatoes, onion, cucumber, olives, parsley, oregano, mint, feta cheese, and red wine vinegar, and toss lightly. Cover and let rest in the refrigerator for at least 30 minutes. Taste the salsa before serving and add a pinch of salt or extra herbs if desired.

2. **Cooking.** To cook the chicken, heat the remaining 1 tablespoon of olive oil in a large nonstick skillet over medium-high heat. Add the chicken pieces and cook for 3 to 6 minutes on each side, depending on the thickness. If the chicken sticks to the pan, it's not quite ready to flip.
When chicken is cooked through, top with the salsa and serve.

Sautéed Chicken Cutlets with Romesco Sauce

PREP TIME: 10 MINUTES / COOK TIME: 5 MINUTES/ SERVES 4

Ingredients

½ slice hearty white sandwich bread, cut into ½ inch pieces
¼ cup hazelnuts, toasted and skinned
2 tablespoons extra-virgin olive oil
2 garlic cloves, sliced thin
1 cup jarred roasted red peppers, rinsed and patted dry
1½ tablespoons sherry vinegar
1 teaspoon honey
½ teaspoon smoked paprika
½ teaspoon salt
Pinch cayenne pepper
4 (4- to 6-ounce) boneless, skinless chicken breasts, trimmed
Salt and pepper
4 teaspoons extra-virgin olive oil

Directions

Preparing the Ingredients

1. For the sauce Cook bread, hazelnuts, and 1 tablespoon oil in 12-inch skillet over medium heat, stirring constantly, until bread and hazelnuts are lightly toasted, about 3 minutes. Add garlic and cook, stirring constantly, until fragrant, about 30 seconds. Transfer mixture to food processor and pulse until coarsely chopped, about 5 pulses. Add red peppers, vinegar, honey, paprika, salt, cayenne, and remaining 1 tablespoon oil to processor. Pulse until finely chopped, 5 to 8 pulses. Transfer sauce to bowl and set aside for serving. (Sauce can be refrigerated for up to 2 days.)

2. For the chicken: Cut chicken horizontally into 2 thin cutlets, then cover with plastic wrap and pound to uniform ¼-inch thickness. Pat cutlets dry with paper towels and season with salt and pepper. Heat 2 teaspoons oil in 12-inch skillet over medium-high heat until just smoking. Place 4 cutlets in skillet and cook, without moving, until browned on first side, about 2 minutes. Flip cutlets and continue to cook until opaque on second side, about 30 seconds. Transfer chicken to serving platter and tent loosely with aluminum foil. Repeat with remaining 4 cutlets and remaining 2 teaspoons oil. Serve with sauce.

3. Sautéed Chicken Cutlets with Sun-Dried Tomato Sauce FAST
Omit honey, smoked paprika, and cayenne. Substitute ¼ cup pine nuts for hazelnuts, 1 small tomato, cored and cut into ½-inch pieces, and ½ cup oil-packed sun-dried tomatoes for red peppers, and 2 tablespoons balsamic vinegar for sherry vinegar. Add 2 tablespoons chopped fresh basil to food processor with tomato.

4. Sautéed Chicken Cutlets with Olive-Orange Sauce FAST
Omit smoked paprika and cayenne. Cut away peel and pith from 1 orange. Quarter orange, then slice crosswise into ½-inch-thick pieces. Substitute ¼ cup slivered almonds for hazelnuts, orange pieces and ¾ cup pitted kalamata olives for red peppers, and 1½ tablespoons red wine vinegar for sherry vinegar. Add ¼ teaspoon fennel seeds to skillet with garlic and 2 tablespoons chopped fresh mint to food processor with orange.

Za'atar Rubbed Chicken with Celery Root and Spinach (Instant Pot)

PREP TIME: 22 MINUTES / COOK TIME: 5 MINUTES/ SERVES 4

Ingredients

2 (12-ounce) bone-in split chicken breasts, skin removed, trimmed
2 teaspoons za'atar
¾ teaspoon table salt, divided
2 pounds celery root, peeled, halved, and sliced ¾ inch thick
1 tablespoon extra-virgin olive oil
¼ teaspoon pepper
½ cup chicken broth
10 ounces (10 cups) baby spinach
½ teaspoon grated lemon zest
¼ cup pomegranate seeds
3 tablespoons coarsely chopped fresh mint
¼ cup Tahini Sauce

Directions

1.　Pat chicken dry with paper towels and sprinkle with za'atar and ½ teaspoon salt. Toss celery root with oil, remaining ¼ teaspoon salt, and pepper in bowl. Add broth to Instant Pot. Place chicken skinned side up in pot, then arrange celery root slabs on top. Lock lid in place and close pressure release valve. Select high pressure cook function and cook for 5 minutes.

2.　Turn off Instant Pot and quick-release pressure. Carefully remove lid, allowing steam to escape away from you. Transfer celery root to serving dish and chicken to cutting board. Tent both with aluminum foil and let rest while preparing spinach.

3.　Add spinach, 1 handful at a time, to cooking liquid left in pot and cook using highest sauté function until wilted and tender, about 2 minutes. Stir in lemon zest and season with salt and pepper to taste. Using tongs, transfer spinach to serving dish with celery root. Sprinkle with pomegranate seeds and mint. Carve chicken from bones and slice ½ inch thick. Serve with vegetables, passing Tahini Sauce separately.

Grilled Oregano Chicken Kebabs with Zucchini and Olives

PREP TIME: 10 MINUTES / COOK TIME: 20 MINUTES/ SERVES 4

Ingredients

Nonstick cooking spray
¼ cup extra-virgin olive oil
2 tablespoons balsamic vinegar
1 teaspoon dried oregano, crushed between your fingers
1pound boneless, skinless chicken breasts, cut into 1½-inch pieces
2 medium zucchini, cut into 1-inch pieces (about 2½ cups)
½ cup Kalamata olives, pitted and halved
2 tablespoons olive brine
¼ cup torn fresh basil leaves

Directions

Preparing the Ingredients

1.　Coat the cold grill with nonstick cooking spray. Heat the grill to medium-high.

In a small bowl, whisk together the oil, vinegar, and oregano. Divide the marinade between two large plastic zip-top bags.

Add the chicken to one bag and the zucchini to another. Seal and massage the marinade into both the chicken and zucchini.

2.　Thread the chicken onto 6 (12-inch) wooden skewers. Thread the zucchini onto 8 or 9 (12-inch) wooden skewers. Cook the kebabs in batches on the grill for 5 minutes, flip, and grill for 5 minutes more, until any chicken juices run clear.

3.　Remove the chicken and zucchini from the skewers and put in a large serving bowl. Toss with the olives, olive brine, and basil and serve.

Crispy Mediterranean Chicken Thighs

PREP TIME: 5 MINUTES / COOK TIME: 30 TO 35 MINUTES/ SERVES 4

Ingredients

2 tablespoons extra-virgin olive oil
2 teaspoons dried rosemary
1½ teaspoons ground cumin
1½ teaspoons ground coriander
¾ teaspoon dried oregano
⅛ teaspoon salt
6 bone-in, skin-on chicken thighs (about 3 pounds)

Directions

Preparing the Ingredients

1.　Preheat the oven to 450°F. Line a baking sheet with parchment paper.

Place the olive oil and spices into a large bowl and mix together, making a paste. Add the chicken and mix together until evenly coated. Place on the prepared baking sheet.

2.　Bake for 30 to 35 minutes, or until golden brown and the chicken registers an internal temperature of 165°F.

To decrease overall saturated fat in the dish, remove the chicken skin prior to mixing with the spices. The finished chicken will still be flavorful, but without a crispy skin.

To add a bit of brightness to the dish, serve with lemon wedges or squeeze half a lemon over the chicken thighs before serving.

Pollock with Roasted Tomatoes

PREP TIME: 5 MINUTES / COOK TIME: 40 MINUTES/ MAKES ¼ CUP / SERVES 6

Ingredients

12 plum tomatoes, halved
2 shallots, very thinly cut into rings
3 garlic cloves, minced
3 tablespoons plus 1 teaspoon extra-virgin olive oil, divided
1 teaspoon sea salt, divided
½ teaspoon freshly ground black pepper, divided
1 teaspoon butter (or extra-virgin olive oil)
¾ cup whole-wheat bread crumbs
6 (4-ounce) pollock fillets
¼ cup chopped fresh Italian parsley leaves

Directions

1.   Preparing the Ingredients

Preheat the oven to 450°F. In a large bowl, toss the tomatoes, shallots, and garlic with 1 tablespoon of olive oil, ½ teaspoon of sea salt, and ¼ teaspoon of pepper. Transfer to a rimmed baking sheet and arrange in a single layer.

2.   Cooking

Bake for about 40 minutes until the tomatoes are soft and browned.

While the tomatoes cook, in a large nonstick skillet over medium-high heat, heat 1 tablespoon plus 1 teaspoon of olive oil until it bubbles. Add the bread crumbs and cook for about 5 minutes, stirring, until they are browned and crunchy. Remove from the pan and set aside, scraping the pan clean. Return the skillet to medium-high heat and add the remaining tablespoon of olive oil. Season the fish with the remaining ½ teaspoon of sea salt and ¼ teaspoon of pepper. Place the fish in the skillet. Cook for about 5 minutes per side until opaque.

To assemble, spoon the tomatoes onto four plates. Top with the pollock and sprinkle with the bread crumbs.

Garnish with parsley and serve. If you can't find pollock, use any white-fleshed fish, such as cod or halibut. If you'd like to cut the saturated fat from this recipe, use olive oil instead of butter.

Greek Yogurt–Marinated Chicken Breasts

PREP TIME: 15 MINUTES, PLUS 30 MINUTES TO MARINATE / COOK TIME: 30 MINUTES/ SERVES 2

Ingredients

½ cup plain Greek yogurt
3 garlic cloves, minced
2 tablespoons minced fresh oregano (or 1 tablespoon dried oregano)
Zest of 1 lemon
1 tablespoon olive oil
½ teaspoon salt
2 (4-ounce) boneless, skinless chicken breasts

Directions

1.   Preparing the Ingredients

In a medium bowl, add the yogurt, garlic, oregano, lemon zest, olive oil, and salt and stir to combine. If the yogurt is very thick, you may need to add a few tablespoons of water or a squeeze of lemon juice to thin it a bit.

Add the chicken to the bowl and toss it in the marinade to coat it well.

Cover and refrigerate the chicken for at least 30 minutes or up to overnight.

Preheat the oven to 350°F and set the rack to the middle position.

2.   Cooking

Place the chicken in a baking dish and roast for 30 minutes, or until chicken reaches an internal temperature of 165°F. Yogurt makes a great base for any marinade flavor.

Just combine it with your favorite fresh or dried herbs or spices.

Honey Almond–Crusted Chicken Tenders

PREP TIME: 10 MINUTES / COOK TIME: 20 MINUTES/ SERVES 4

Ingredients

Nonstick cooking spray
1 tablespoon honey
1 tablespoon whole-grain or Dijon mustard
¼ teaspoon kosher or sea salt
¼ teaspoon freshly ground black pepper
1pound boneless, skinless chicken breast tenders or tenderloins
1 cup almonds (about 3 ounces)

Directions

1.   Preparing the Ingredients

Preheat the oven to 425°F. Line a large, rimmed baking sheet with parchment paper. Place a wire cooling rack on the parchment-lined baking sheet, and coat the rack well with nonstick cooking spray. In a large bowl, combine the honey, mustard, salt, and pepper. Add the chicken and stir gently to coat. Set aside.

Use a knife or a mini food processor to roughly chop the almonds; they should be about the size of sunflower seeds. Dump the nuts onto a large sheet of parchment paper and spread them out. Press the coated chicken tenders into the nuts until evenly coated on all sides. Place the chicken on the prepared wire rack.

2.   Cooking.

Bake for 15 to 20 minutes, or until the internal temperature of the chicken measures 165°F on a meat thermometer and any juices run clear. Serve immediately.

Greek Turkey Burger

PREP TIME: 10 MINUTES / COOK TIME: 10 MINUTES/ SERVES 4

Ingredients

1 pound ground turkey
1 medium zucchini, grated
¼ cup whole-wheat bread crumbs
¼ cup red onion, minced
¼ cup crumbled feta cheese
1 large egg, beaten
1 garlic clove, minced
1 tablespoon fresh oregano, chopped
1 teaspoon kosher salt
¼ teaspoon freshly ground black pepper
1 tablespoon extra-virgin olive oil

Directions

1.   Preparing the Ingredients

In a large bowl, combine the turkey, zucchini, bread crumbs, onion, feta cheese, egg, garlic, oregano, salt, and black pepper, and mix well. Shape into 4 equal patties.

2.   Cooking

Heat the olive oil in a large nonstick grill pan or skillet over medium-high heat. Add the burgers to the pan and reduce the heat to medium. Cook on one side for 5 minutes, then flip and cook the other side for 5 minutes more.

Any summer squash can be used in this recipe, so feel free to swap out the zucchini for yellow squash or pattypan squash.

Turkey Burgers with Mango Salsa

PREP TIME: 15 MINUTES / COOK TIME: 10 MINUTES/ SERVES 6

Ingredients

1½ pounds ground turkey breast
1 teaspoon sea salt, divided
¼ teaspoon freshly ground black pepper
2 tablespoons extra-virgin olive oil
2 mangos, peeled, pitted, and cubed
½ red onion, finely chopped
Juice of 1 lime
1 garlic clove, minced
½ jalapeño pepper, seeded and finely minced
2 tablespoons chopped fresh cilantro leaves

Directions

1.   Preparing the Ingredients

Form the turkey breast into 4 patties and season with ½ teaspoon of sea salt and the pepper.

In a large nonstick skillet over medium-high heat, heat the olive oil until it shimmers.

2.   Cooking

Add the turkey patties and cook for about 5 minutes per side until browned.

While the patties cook, mix together the mango, red onion, lime juice, garlic, jalapeño, cilantro, and remaining ½ teaspoon of sea salt in a small bowl.

Spoon the salsa over the turkey patties and serve.

Serve this salsa over grilled halibut. Heat the grill to medium-high heat and brush it with olive oil. Grill 4 (4- to 6-ounce) halibut fillets for about 6 minutes per side. Top with the salsa.

Bruschetta Chicken Burgers

PREP TIME: 15 MINUTES / COOK TIME: 15 MINUTES/ SERVES 2

Ingredients

1 tablespoon olive oil
3 tablespoons finely minced onion
2 garlic cloves, minced
1 teaspoon dried basil
¼ teaspoon salt
3 tablespoons minced sun-dried tomatoes packed in olive oil
8 ounces ground chicken breast
3 pieces small mozzarella balls (ciliegine), minced

Directions

Preparing the Ingredients

**1.   **Heat the grill to high heat (about 400°F) and oil the grill grates. Alternatively, you can cook these in a nonstick skillet.

Heat the olive oil in a small skillet over medium-high heat. Add the onion and garlic and sauté for 5 minutes, until softened. Stir in the basil. Remove from the heat and place in a medium bowl.

Add the salt, sun-dried tomatoes, and ground chicken and stir to combine. Mix in the mozzarella balls. Divide the chicken mixture in half and form into two burgers, each about ¾-inch thick.

**2.   **Place the burgers on the grill and cook for five minutes, or until golden on the bottom.

Flip the burgers over and grill for another five minutes, or until they reach an internal temperature of 165°F.

**3.   **If cooking the burgers in a skillet on the stovetop, heat a nonstick skillet over medium-high heat and add the burgers. Cook them for 5 to 6 minutes on the first side, or until golden brown on the bottom. Flip the burgers and cook for an additional 5 minutes, or until they reach an internal temperature of 165°F.

If you're not in the mood for burgers, form the chicken mixture into small meatballs and eat them with tomato sauce and pasta. Panfry them or bake them in the oven at 350°F for 15 to 20 minutes.

Chicken and Spiced Freekeh with Cilantro and Preserved Lemon (Instant Pot)

PREP TIME: 30 MINUTES / COOK TIME: 5 MINUTES/ SERVES 4

Ingredients

2 tablespoons extra-virgin olive oil, plus extra for drizzling
1 onion, chopped fine
4 garlic cloves, minced
1½ teaspoons smoked paprika
¼ teaspoon ground cardamom
¼ teaspoon red pepper flakes
2¼ cups chicken broth
1½ cups cracked freekeh, rinsed
2 (12-ounce) bone-in split chicken breasts, halved crosswise and trimmed
½ teaspoon table salt
¼ teaspoon pepper
¼ cup chopped fresh cilantro
2 tablespoons sesame seeds, toasted
½ preserved lemon, pulp and white pith removed, rind rinsed and minced (2 tablespoons)

Directions

**1.   **Using highest sauté function, heat oil in Instant Pot until shimmering. Add onion and cook until softened, about 5 minutes. Stir in garlic, paprika, cardamom, and pepper flakes and cook until fragrant, about 30 seconds. Stir in broth and freekeh. Sprinkle chicken with salt and pepper. Nestle skin side up into freekeh mixture. Lock lid in place and close pressure release valve. Select high pressure cook function and cook for 5 minutes.

**2.   **Turn off Instant Pot and quick-release pressure. Carefully remove lid, allowing steam to escape away from you. Transfer chicken to serving

dish and discard skin, if desired. Tent with aluminum foil and let rest while finishing freekeh.
3.   Gently fluff freekeh with fork. Lay clean dish towel over pot, replace lid, and let sit for 5 minutes. Season with salt and pepper to taste. Transfer freekeh to serving dish with chicken and sprinkle with cilantro, sesame seeds, and preserved lemon. Drizzle with extra oil and serve.

One-Pan Parsley Chicken and Potatoes

PREP TIME: 5 MINUTES / COOK TIME: 25 MINUTES/ SERVES 6
Ingredients
1½ pounds boneless, skinless chicken thighs, cut into 1-inch cubes
1 tablespoon extra-virgin olive oil
1½ pounds Yukon Gold potatoes, unpeeled, cut into ½-inch cubes (about 6 small potatoes)
2 garlic cloves, minced (about 1 teaspoon)
¼ cup dry white wine or apple cider vinegar
1 cup low-sodium or no-salt-added chicken broth
1 tablespoon Dijon mustard
¼ teaspoon kosher or sea salt
¼ teaspoon freshly ground black pepper
1 cup chopped fresh flat-leaf (Italian) parsley, including stems
1 tablespoon freshly squeezed lemon juice (½ small lemon)
Directions
1.   **Preparing the Ingredients**. Pat the chicken dry with a few paper towels. In a large skillet over medium-high heat, heat the oil.
2.   **Cooking**. Add the chicken and cook for 5 minutes, stirring only after the chicken has browned on one side. Remove the chicken from the pan with a slotted spoon, and put it on a plate; it will not yet be fully cooked. Leave the skillet on the stove.
Add the potatoes to the skillet and cook for 5 minutes, stirring only after the potatoes have become golden and crispy on one side. Push the potatoes to the side of the skillet, add the garlic, and cook, stirring constantly, for 1 minute. Add the wine and cook for 1 minute, until nearly evaporated. Add the chicken broth, mustard, salt, pepper, and reserved chicken pieces. Turn the heat up to high, and bring to a boil. Once boiling, cover the skillet, reduce the heat to medium-low, and cook for 10 to 12 minutes, until the potatoes are tender and the internal temperature of the chicken measures 165°F on a meat thermometer and any juices run clear. During the last minute of cooking, stir in the parsley. Remove from the heat, stir in the lemon juice, and serve.

Harissa Yogurt Chicken Thighs

PREP TIME: 5 MINUTES, PLUS 15 MINUTES TO MARINATE / COOK TIME: 25 MINUTES/ SERVES 4
Ingredients
½ cup plain Greek yogurt
2 tablespoons harissa
1 tablespoon lemon juice
½ teaspoon kosher salt
¼ teaspoon freshly ground black pepper
1½ pounds boneless, skinless chicken thighs
Directions
1.   **Preparing the Ingredients**
In a bowl, combine the yogurt, harissa, lemon juice, salt, and black pepper. Add the chicken and mix together. Marinate for at least 15 minutes, and up to 4 hours in the refrigerator.
2.   **Cooking**
Preheat the oven to 425°F. Line a baking sheet with parchment paper or foil. Remove the chicken thighs from the marinade and arrange in a single layer on the baking sheet. Roast for 20 minutes, turning the chicken over halfway.
Change the oven temperature to broil. Broil the chicken until golden brown in spots, 2 to 3 minutes.

Herb-Roasted Turkey Breast

PREP TIME: 15 MINUTES / COOK TIME: 1½ HOURS (PLUS 20 MINUTES TO REST)/ SERVES 6
Ingredients
2 tablespoons extra-virgin olive oil
4 garlic cloves, minced
Zest of 1 lemon
1 tablespoon chopped fresh thyme leaves
1 tablespoon chopped fresh rosemary leaves
2 tablespoons chopped fresh Italian parsley leaves
1 teaspoon ground mustard
1 teaspoon sea salt
¼ teaspoon freshly ground black pepper
1 (6-pound) bone-in, skin-on turkey breast
1 cup dry white wine
Directions
1.   **Preparing the Ingredients**
Preheat the oven to 325°F.
In a small bowl, whisk the olive oil, garlic, lemon zest, thyme, rosemary, parsley, mustard, sea salt, and pepper. Spread the herb mixture evenly over the surface of the turkey breast, and loosen the skin and rub underneath as well. Place the turkey breast in a roasting pan on a rack, skin-side up.
2.   **Cooking**.
Pour the wine in the pan. Roast for 1 to 1½ hours until the turkey reaches an internal temperature of 165°F. Remove from the oven and let rest for 20 minutes, tented with aluminum foil to keep it warm, before carving.

Chicken Gyros with Grilled Vegetables and Tzatziki Sauce

PREP TIME: 15 MINUTES, PLUS 30 MINUTES TO MARINATE / COOK TIME: 15 MINUTES/ SERVES 2
Ingredients
2 tablespoons freshly squeezed lemon juice
2 tablespoons olive oil, divided, plus extra for oiling the grill
1 teaspoon minced fresh oregano, or ½ teaspoon dry oregano
½ teaspoon garlic powder

½ teaspoon salt, divided, plus more to season vegetables
8 ounces chicken tenders
1 small zucchini, cut into ½-inch strips lengthwise
1 small eggplant, cut into 1-inch strips lengthwise
½ red pepper, seeded and cut in half lengthwise
¾ cup plain Greek yogurt
½ English cucumber, peeled and minced
1 tablespoon minced fresh dill
2 (8-inch) pita breads

Directions

1.   Preparing the Ingredients

In a medium bowl, combine the lemon juice, 1 tablespoon of olive oil, the oregano, garlic powder, and ¼ teaspoon of salt. Add the chicken and marinate for 30 minutes.

Place the zucchini, eggplant, and red pepper in a large mixing bowl and sprinkle liberally with salt and the remaining 1 tablespoon of olive oil. Toss them well to coat. Let the vegetables rest while the chicken is marinating.

In a medium bowl, combine the yogurt, the cucumber, the remaining salt, and the dill. Stir well to combine and set aside in the refrigerator.

When ready to grill, heat the grill to medium-high (350–400°F) and oil the grill grate.

Drain any liquid from the vegetables and place them on the grill. Remove the chicken tenders from the marinade and place them on the grill.

2.   Cooking

Cook chicken and vegetables for 3 minutes per side, or until the chicken is no longer pink inside and the vegetables have grill marks.

Remove the chicken and vegetables from the grill and set aside. On the grill, heat the pitas for about 30 seconds, flipping them frequently so they don't burn. Divide the chicken tenders and vegetables between the pitas and top each with ¼ cup of the tzatziki sauce. Roll the pitas up like a cone to eat.

This is also great if you grill the chicken and vegetables ahead of time and enjoy it cold. You can also vary the vegetables: Try a portobello mushroom, sweet onion slices, or summer squash.

Braised Chicken with Mushrooms and Tomatoes (Instant Pot)

PREP TIME: 30 MINUTES / COOK TIME: 15 MINUTES/ SERVES 4

Ingredients

1 tablespoon extra-virgin olive oil
1pound portobello mushroom caps, gills removed, caps halved and sliced ½ inch thick
1 onion, chopped fine
¾ teaspoon salt, divided
4 garlic cloves, minced
1 tablespoon tomato paste
1 tablespoon all-purpose flour
2 teaspoons minced fresh sage
½ cup dry red wine
1 (14.5-ounce) can diced tomatoes, drained

4 (5- to 7-ounce) bone-in chicken thighs, skin removed, trimmed
¼ teaspoon pepper
2 tablespoons chopped fresh parsley
Shaved Parmesan cheese

Directions

1.   Using highest sauté function, heat oil in Instant Pot until shimmering. Add mushrooms, onion, and ¼ teaspoon salt. Partially cover and cook until mushrooms are softened and have released their liquid, about 5 minutes. Stir in garlic, tomato paste, flour, and sage and cook until fragrant, about 1 minute. Stir in wine, scraping up any browned bits, then stir in tomatoes.

2.   Sprinkle chicken with remaining ½ teaspoon salt and pepper. Nestle chicken skinned side up into pot and spoon some of sauce on top. Lock lid in place and close pressure release valve. Select high pressure cook function and cook for 15 minutes.

3.   Turn off Instant Pot and quick-release pressure. Carefully remove lid, allowing steam to escape away from you. Transfer chicken to serving dish, tent with aluminum foil, and let rest while finishing sauce.

4.   Using highest sauté function, bring sauce to simmer and cook until thickened slightly, about 5 minutes. Season sauce with salt and pepper to taste. Spoon sauce over chicken and sprinkle with parsley and Parmesan.

Sumac Chicken with Cauliflower and Carrots

PREP TIME: 15 MINUTES / COOK TIME: 40 MINUTES/ SERVES 4

Ingredients

3 tablespoons extra-virgin olive oil
1 tablespoon ground sumac
1 teaspoon kosher salt
½ teaspoon ground cumin
¼ teaspoon freshly ground black pepper
1½ pounds bone-in chicken thighs and drumsticks
1 medium cauliflower, cut into 1-inch florets
2 carrots, peeled and cut into 1-inch rounds
1 lemon, cut into ¼-inch-thick slices
1 tablespoon lemon juice
¼ cup fresh parsley, chopped
¼ cup fresh mint, chopped

Directions

1.   Preparing the Ingredients

Preheat the oven to 425°F. Line a baking sheet with parchment paper or foil.

In a large bowl, whisk together the olive oil, sumac, salt, cumin, and black pepper. Add the chicken, cauliflower, and carrots and toss until thoroughly coated with the oil and spice mixture.

Arrange the cauliflower, carrots, and chicken in a single layer on the baking sheet. Top with the lemon slices.

2.   Cooking

Roast for 40 minutes, tossing the vegetables once halfway through. Sprinkle the lemon juice over the chicken and vegetables and garnish with the parsley and mint.

Chicken Sausage and Peppers

PREP TIME: 10 MINUTES / COOK TIME: 20 MINUTES / SERVES 6

Ingredients

2 tablespoons extra-virgin olive oil
6 Italian chicken sausage links
1 onion, thinly sliced
1 red bell pepper, seeded and thinly sliced
1 green bell pepper, seeded and thinly sliced
3 garlic cloves, minced
½ cup dry white wine
½ teaspoon sea salt
¼ teaspoon freshly ground black pepper
Pinch red pepper flakes

Directions

Preparing the Ingredients

1.	In a large skillet over medium-high heat, heat the olive oil until it shimmers. Add the sausages and cook for 5 to 7 minutes, turning occasionally, until browned, and they reach an internal temperature of 165°F. With tongs, remove the sausage from the pan and set aside on a platter, tented with aluminum foil to keep warm.

2.	Return the skillet to the heat and add the onion, red bell pepper, and green bell pepper. Cook for 5 to 7 minutes, stirring occasionally, until the vegetables begin to brown. Add the garlic and cook for 30 seconds, stirring constantly.

Stir in the wine, sea salt, pepper, and red pepper flakes. Use the side of a spoon to scrape and fold in any browned bits from the bottom of the pan. Simmer for about 4 minutes more, stirring, until the liquid reduces by half. Spoon the peppers over the sausages and serve.

Skillet Greek Turkey and Rice

PREP TIME: 20 MINUTES / COOK TIME: 30 MINUTES / SERVES 2

Ingredients

1 tablespoon olive oil
½ medium onion, minced
2 garlic cloves, minced
8 ounces ground turkey breast
½ cup roasted red peppers, chopped (about 2 jarred peppers)
¼ cup sun-dried tomatoes, minced
1 teaspoon dried oregano
½ cup brown rice
1¼ cups low-sodium chicken stock
Salt
2 cups lightly packed baby spinach

Directions

Preparing the Ingredients

1.	Heat the olive oil in a sauté pan over medium heat. Add the onion and sauté for 5 minutes.

Add the garlic and cook for another 30 seconds. Add the turkey breast and cook for 7 minutes, breaking the turkey up with a spoon, until no longer pink. Add the roasted red peppers, sun-dried tomatoes, and oregano and stir to combine. Add the rice and chicken stock and bring the mixture to a boil.

2.	Cover the pan and reduce the heat to medium-low. Simmer for 30 minutes, or until the rice is cooked and tender. Season with salt. Add the spinach to the pan and stir until it wilts slightly.

Chicken Tagine (Instant Pot)

PREP TIME: 30 MINUTES / COOK TIME: 10 MINUTES / SERVES 4

Ingredients

2 (15-ounce) cans chickpeas, rinsed, divided
1 tablespoon extra-virgin olive oil
5 garlic cloves, minced
1½ teaspoons paprika
½ teaspoon ground turmeric
½ teaspoon ground cumin
¼ teaspoon ground ginger
¼ teaspoon cayenne pepper
1 fennel bulb, 1 tablespoon fronds minced, stalks discarded, bulb halved and cut lengthwise into ½-inch-thick wedges
1 cup chicken broth
3 (2-inch) strips lemon zest, plus lemon wedges for serving
4 (5- to 7-ounce) bone-in chicken thighs, skin removed, trimmed
½ teaspoon table salt
½ cup pitted large brine-cured green or black olives, halved
⅓ cup raisins
2 tablespoons chopped fresh parsley

Directions

1.	Using potato masher, mash ½ cup chickpeas in bowl to paste. Using highest sauté function, cook oil, garlic, paprika, turmeric, cumin, ginger, and cayenne in Instant Pot until fragrant, about 1 minute. Turn off Instant Pot, then stir in remaining whole chickpeas, mashed chickpeas, fennel wedges, broth, and zest.

2.	Sprinkle chicken with salt. Nestle chicken skinned side up into pot and spoon some of cooking liquid over top. Lock lid in place and close pressure release valve. Select high pressure cook function and cook for 10 minutes.

3.	Turn off Instant Pot and quick-release pressure. Carefully remove lid, allowing steam to escape away from you. Discard lemon zest. Stir in olives, raisins, parsley, and fennel fronds. Season with salt and pepper to taste. Serve with lemon wedges.

Lemon Chicken with Artichokes and Crispy Kale

PREP TIME: 15 MINUTES, PLUS 30 MINUTES TO MARINATE / COOK TIME: 35 MINUTES / SERVES 4

Ingredients

3 tablespoons extra-virgin olive oil, divided
2 tablespoons lemon juice
Zest of 1 lemon
2 garlic cloves, minced
2 teaspoons dried rosemary
½ teaspoon kosher salt
¼ teaspoon freshly ground black pepper
1½ pounds boneless, skinless chicken breast
2 (14-ounce) cans artichoke hearts, drained
1 bunch (about 6 ounces) lacinato kale, stemmed and torn or chopped into pieces

Directions

1.   Preparing the Ingredients

In a large bowl or zip-top bag, combine 2 tablespoons of the olive oil, the lemon juice, lemon zest, garlic, rosemary, salt, and black pepper. Mix well and then add the chicken and artichokes. Marinate for at least 30 minutes, and up to 4 hours in the refrigerator.

2.   Cooking

Preheat the oven to 350°F. Line a baking sheet with parchment paper or foil. Remove the chicken and artichokes from the marinade and spread them in a single layer on the baking sheet. Roast for 15 minutes, turn the chicken over, and roast another 15 minutes. Remove the baking sheet and put the chicken, artichokes, and juices on a platter or large plate. Tent with foil to keep warm. Change the oven temperature to broil. In a large bowl, combine the kale with the remaining 1 tablespoon of the olive oil. Arrange the kale on the baking sheet and broil until golden brown in spots and as crispy as you like, about 3 to 5 minutes. Place the kale on top of the chicken and artichokes.

Chicken Piccata

PREP TIME: 10 MINUTES / COOK TIME: 15 MINUTES / SERVES 6

Ingredients

½ cup whole-wheat flour
½ teaspoon sea salt
⅛ teaspoon freshly ground black pepper
1½ pounds boneless, skinless chicken breasts, cut into 6 pieces and pounded ½-inch thick
3 tablespoons extra-virgin olive oil
1 cup unsalted chicken broth
½ cup dry white wine
Juice of 1 lemon
Zest of 1 lemon
¼ cup capers, drained and rinsed
¼ cup chopped fresh parsley leaves

Directions

1.   Preparing the Ingredients

In a shallow dish, whisk the flour, sea salt, and pepper. Dredge the chicken in the flour and tap off any excess. In a large skillet over medium-high heat, heat the olive oil until it shimmers.

2.   Cooking

Add the chicken and cook for about 4 minutes per side until browned. Remove the chicken from the pan

and set aside, tented with aluminum foil to keep warm. Return the skillet to the heat and add the broth, wine, lemon juice, and lemon zest, and capers. Use the side of a spoon to scrape and fold in any browned bits from the bottom of the pan.
Simmer for 3 to 4 minutes, stirring, until the liquid thickens. Remove the skillet from the heat and return the chicken to the pan. Turn to coat. Stir in the parsley and serve.
To pound the chicken to an even thickness: Place the chicken between two pieces of plastic wrap or parchment paper and use a flat kitchen mallet or a smooth-bottomed heavy saucepan to pound until they reach the desired thickness. Use caution to avoid puncturing the plastic or paper.

Lemon and Paprika Herb-Marinated Chicken

PREP TIME: 10 MINUTES, PLUS 30 MINUTES TO MARINATE / COOK TIME: 15 MINUTES/ SERVES 2

Ingredients

2 tablespoons olive oil
4 tablespoons freshly squeezed lemon juice
¼ teaspoon salt
1 teaspoon paprika
1 teaspoon dried basil
½ teaspoon dried thyme
¼ teaspoon garlic powder
2 (4-ounce) boneless, skinless chicken breasts

Directions

1.   Preparing the Ingredients

In a bowl with a lid, combine the olive oil, lemon juice, salt, paprika, basil, thyme, and garlic powder.
Add the chicken and marinate for at least 30 minutes, or up to 4 hours.

2.   Cooking

When ready to cook, heat the grill to medium-high (about 350–400°F) and oil the grill grate. Alternately, you can also cook these in a nonstick sauté pan over medium-high heat.
Grill the chicken for 6 to 7 minutes, or until it lifts away from the grill easily. Flip it over and grill for another 6 to 7 minutes, or until it reaches an internal temperature of 165°F.
When grilling (or panfrying) chicken breasts, don't disturb them for a few minutes. If they don't lift off the grill easily, they're not done yet!

Tahini Chicken Rice Bowls

PREP TIME: 10 MINUTES / COOK TIME: 15 MINUTES / SERVES 4

Ingredients

1 cup uncooked instant brown rice
¼ cup tahini or peanut butter (tahini for nut-free)
¼ cup 2% plain Greek yogurt
2 tablespoons chopped scallions, green and white parts (2 scallions)
1 tablespoon freshly squeezed lemon juice (from ½ medium lemon)
1 tablespoon water

1 teaspoon ground cumin
¾ teaspoon ground cinnamon
¼ teaspoon kosher or sea salt
2 cups chopped cooked chicken breast (about 1 pound)
½ cup chopped dried apricots
2 cups peeled and chopped seedless cucumber (1 large cucumber)
4 teaspoons sesame seeds
Fresh mint leaves, for serving (optional)
Directions
Preparing the Ingredients
1.	Cook the brown rice according to the package instructions.While the rice is cooking, in a medium bowl, mix together the tahini, yogurt, scallions, lemon juice, water, cumin, cinnamon, and salt. Transfer half the tahini mixture to another medium bowl. Mix the chicken into the first bowl.When the rice is done, mix it into the second bowl of tahini (the one without the chicken).
2.	To assemble, divide the chicken among four bowls. Spoon the rice mixture next to the chicken in each bowl. Next to the chicken, place the dried apricots, and in the remaining empty section, add the cucumbers. Sprinkle with sesame seeds, and top with mint, if desired, and serve.

Za'atar Chicken Tenders

PREP TIME: 5 MINUTES / COOK TIME: 15 MINUTES/ SERVES 4
Ingredients
Olive oil cooking spray
1 pound chicken tenders
1½ tablespoons za'atar
½ teaspoon kosher salt
¼ teaspoon freshly ground black pepper
Directions
Preparing the Ingredients Preheat the oven to 450°F. Line a baking sheet with parchment paper or foil and lightly spray with olive oil cooking spray. In a large bowl, combine the chicken, za'atar, salt, and black pepper. Mix together well, covering the chicken tenders fully. Arrange in a single layer on the baking sheet and bake for 15 minutes, turning the chicken over once halfway through the cooking time.

One-Pan Tuscan Chicken

PREP TIME: 10 MINUTES / COOK TIME: 25 MINUTES/ SERVES 6
Ingredients
¼ cup extra-virgin olive oil, divided
1 pound boneless, skinless chicken breasts, cut into ¾-inch pieces
1 onion, chopped
1 red bell pepper, chopped
3 garlic cloves, minced
½ cup dry white wine
1 (14-ounce) can crushed tomatoes, undrained
1 (14-ounce) can chopped tomatoes, drained
1 (14-ounce) can white beans, drained

1 tablespoon dried Italian seasoning
½ teaspoon sea salt
⅛ teaspoon freshly ground black pepper
⅛ teaspoon red pepper flakes
¼ cup chopped fresh basil leaves
Directions
Preparing the Ingredients
1.	In a large skillet over medium-high heat, heat 2 tablespoons of olive oil until it shimmers. Add the chicken and cook for about 6 minutes, stirring, until browned. Remove the chicken from the skillet and set aside on a platter, tented with aluminum foil to keep warm.
2.	Return the skillet to the heat and heat the remaining 2 tablespoons of olive oil until it shimmers. Add the onion and red bell pepper. Cook for about 5 minutes, stirring occasionally, until the vegetables are soft.
Add the garlic and cook for 30 seconds, stirring constantly. Stir in the wine, and use the side of the spoon to scrape and fold in any browned bits from the bottom of the pan. Cook for 1 minute, stirring. Add the crushed and chopped tomatoes, white beans, Italian seasoning, sea salt, pepper, and red pepper flakes. Bring to a simmer and reduce the heat to medium. Cook for 5 minutes, stirring occasionally. Return the chicken and any juices that have collected to the skillet. Cook for 1 to 2 minutes until the chicken heats through. Remove from the heat and stir in the basil before serving. Add ½ cup chopped black or green olives and 1 cup thawed frozen spinach when you return the chicken to the pan.

Skillet Creamy Tarragon Chicken and Mushrooms

PREP TIME: 10 MINUTES / COOK TIME: 20 MINUTES / SERVES 2
Ingredients
2 tablespoons olive oil, divided
½ medium onion, minced
4 ounces baby bella (cremini) mushrooms, sliced
2 small garlic cloves, minced
8 ounces chicken cutlets
2 teaspoons tomato paste
2 teaspoons dried tarragon
2 cups low-sodium chicken stock
6 ounces pappardelle pasta
¼ cup plain full-fat Greek yogurt
Salt
Freshly ground black pepper
Directions
Preparing the Ingredients
1.	Heat 1 tablespoon of the olive oil in a sauté pan over medium-high heat. Add the onion and mushrooms and sauté for 5 minutes. Add the garlic and cook for 1 minute more.
Move the vegetables to the edges of the pan and add the remaining 1 tablespoon of olive oil to the center of the pan. Place the cutlets in the center and let them cook for about 3 minutes, or until they lift up easily

and are golden brown on the bottom. Flip the chicken and cook for another 3 minutes.

Mix in the tomato paste and tarragon. Add the chicken stock and stir well to combine everything. Bring the stock to a boil.

Add the pappardelle. Break up the pasta if needed to fit into the pan. Stir the noodles so they don't stick to the bottom of the pan.

2.   Cover the sauté pan and reduce the heat to medium-low. Let the chicken and noodles simmer for 15 minutes, stirring occasionally, until the pasta is cooked and the liquid is mostly absorbed. If the liquid absorbs too quickly and the pasta isn't cooked, add more water or chicken stock, about ¼ cup at a time as needed.

Remove the pan from the heat.

Stir 2 tablespoons of the hot liquid from the pan into the yogurt. Pour the tempered yogurt into the pan and stir well to mix it into the sauce. Season with salt and pepper.

The sauce will tighten up as it cools, so if it seems too thick, add a few tablespoons of water.

Chicken with Lentils and Butternut Squash (Instant Pot)

PREP TIME: 35 MINUTES / COOK TIME: 15 MINUTES / SERVES 4

Ingredients
2 large shallots, halved and sliced thin, divided
5 teaspoons extra-virgin olive oil, divided
½ teaspoon grated lemon zest plus 2 teaspoons juice
1 teaspoon table salt, divided
4 (5- to 7-ounce) bone-in chicken thighs, trimmed
¼ teaspoon pepper
2 garlic cloves, minced
1½ teaspoons caraway seeds
1 teaspoon ground coriander
1 teaspoon ground cumin
½ teaspoon paprika
⅛ teaspoon cayenne pepper
2 cups chicken broth
1 cup French green lentils, picked over and rinsed
2 pounds butternut squash, peeled, seeded, and cut into 1½-inch pieces (6 cups)
1 cup fresh parsley or cilantro leaves

Directions
1.   Combine half of shallots, 1 tablespoon oil, lemon zest and juice, and ¼ teaspoon salt in bowl; set aside. Pat chicken dry with paper towels and sprinkle with ½ teaspoon salt and pepper. Using highest sauté function, heat remaining 2 teaspoons oil in Instant Pot for 5 minutes (or until just smoking). Place chicken skin side down in pot and cook until well browned on first side, about 5 minutes; transfer to plate.

2.   Add remaining shallot and remaining ¼ teaspoon salt to fat left in pot and cook, using highest sauté function, until shallot is softened, about 2 minutes. Stir in garlic, caraway, coriander, cumin, paprika, and cayenne and cook until fragrant, about

30 seconds. Stir in broth, scraping up any browned bits, then stir in lentils.

Nestle chicken skin side up into lentils and add any accumulated juices. Arrange squash on top. Lock lid in place and close pressure release valve. Select high pressure cook function and cook for 15 minutes.

3.   Turn off Instant Pot and quick-release pressure. Carefully remove lid, allowing steam to escape away from you. Transfer chicken to plate and discard skin, if desired. Season lentil mixture with salt and pepper to taste. Add parsley to shallot mixture and toss to combine. Serve chicken with lentil mixture, topping individual portions with shallot-parsley salad.

Sheet Pan Lemon Chicken and Roasted Artichokes

PREP TIME: 10 MINUTES / COOK TIME: 20 MINUTES/ SERVES 4

Ingredients
2 large lemons
3 tablespoons extra-virgin olive oil, divided
½ teaspoon kosher or sea salt
2 large artichokes
4 (6-ounce) bone-in, skin-on chicken thighs

Directions
Preparing the Ingredients
1.   Put a large, rimmed baking sheet in the oven. Preheat the oven to 450°F with the pan inside. Tear off four sheets of aluminum foil about 8-by-10 inches each; set aside.

2.   Using a Microplane or citrus zester, zest 1 lemon into a large bowl. Halve both lemons and squeeze all the juice into the bowl with the zest. Whisk in 2 tablespoons of oil and the salt. Set aside.

3.   Rinse the artichokes with cool water, and dry with a clean towel. Using a sharp knife, cut about 1½ inches off the tip of each artichoke. Cut about ¼ inch off each stem. Halve each artichoke lengthwise so each piece has equal amounts of stem. Immediately plunge the artichoke halves into the lemon juice and oil mixture (to prevent browning) and turn to coat on all sides. Lay one artichoke half flat-side down in the center of a sheet of aluminum foil, and close up loosely to make a foil packet. Repeat the process with the remaining three artichoke halves. Set the packets aside.

Put the chicken in the remaining lemon juice mixture and turn to coat.

4.   Using oven mitts, carefully remove the hot baking sheet from the oven and pour on the remaining tablespoon of oil; tilt the pan to coat. Carefully arrange the chicken, skin-side down, on the hot baking sheet. Place the artichoke packets, flat-side down, on the baking sheet as well. (Arrange the artichoke packets and chicken with space between them so air can circulate around them.)

5.   Roast for 20 minutes, or until the internal temperature of the chicken measures 165°F on a meat thermometer and any juices run clear. Before

serving, check the artichokes for doneness by pulling on a leaf. If it comes out easily, the artichoke is ready.

Chicken Stew with Artichokes, Capers, and Olives

PREP TIME: 20 MINUTES / COOK TIME: 35 MINUTES / SERVES 4

Ingredients

1½ pounds boneless, skinless chicken thighs
1 teaspoon kosher salt, divided
¼ teaspoon freshly ground black pepper
2 tablespoons olive oil
1 onion, julienned
4 garlic cloves, sliced
1 teaspoon ground turmeric
1 teaspoon ground cumin
½ teaspoon ground coriander
½ teaspoon ground cinnamon
¼ teaspoon red pepper flakes
1 dried bay leaf
1¼ cups no-salt-added chicken stock
¼ cup white wine vinegar
2 tablespoons lemon juice
1 tablespoon lemon zest
1 (14-ounce) can artichoke hearts, drained
¼ cup olives, pitted and chopped
1 teaspoon capers, rinsed and chopped
1 tablespoon fresh mint, chopped
1 tablespoon fresh parsley, chopped

Directions

1.   **Preparing the Ingredients**.
Season the chicken with ½ teaspoon of salt and pepper.

2.   **Cooking.**
Heat the olive oil in a large skillet or sauté pan over medium heat. Add the chicken and sauté 2 to 3 minutes per side. Transfer to a plate and set aside. Add the onion to the same pan and sauté until translucent, about 5 minutes. Add the garlic and sauté 30 seconds. Add the remaining ½ teaspoon salt, the turmeric, cumin, coriander, cinnamon, red pepper flakes, and bay leaf and sauté 30 seconds. Add ¼ cup of the chicken stock and increase the heat to medium-high to deglaze the pan, scraping up any brown bits on the bottom. Add the remaining 1 cup stock, the lemon juice, and lemon zest. Cover, lower the heat to low, and simmer for 10 minutes. Add the artichokes, olives, and capers and mix well. Add the reserved chicken and nestle it into the mixture. Simmer, uncovered, until the chicken fully cooks through, about 10 to 15 minutes. Garnish with the mint and parsley.

BEEF, PORK AND LAMB

Spicy Lamb Burgers with Harissa Mayo

PREP TIME: 15 MINUTES / COOK TIME: 10 MINUTES / SERVES 2

Ingredients
½ small onion, minced
1 garlic clove, minced
2 teaspoons minced fresh parsley
2 teaspoons minced fresh mint
¼ teaspoon salt
Pinch freshly ground black pepper
1 teaspoon cumin
1 teaspoon smoked paprika
¼ teaspoon coriander
8 ounces lean ground lamb
2 tablespoons olive oil mayonnaise
½ teaspoon harissa paste (more or less to taste)
2 hamburger buns or pitas, fresh greens, tomato slices (optional, for serving)

Directions
1. **Preparing the Ingredients**. Preheat the grill to medium-high (350–400°F) and oil the grill grate. Alternatively, you can cook these in a heavy pan (cast iron is best) on the stovetop.
In a large bowl, combine the onion, garlic, parsley, mint, salt, pepper, cumin, paprika, and coriander. Add the lamb and, using your hands, combine the meat with the spices so they are evenly distributed. Form meat mixture into 2 patties.
2. **Cooking**. Grill the burgers for 4 minutes per side, or until the internal temperature registers 160°F for medium.
If cooking on the stovetop, heat the pan to medium-high and oil the pan. Cook the burgers for 5 to 6 minutes per side, or until the internal temperature registers 160°F.
While the burgers are cooking, combine the mayonnaise and harissa in a small bowl.
Serve the burgers with the harissa mayonnaise and slices of tomato and fresh greens on a bun or pita—or skip the bun altogether.
If you don't have harissa available, season your mayonnaise with ½ teaspoon of cumin and ½ teaspoon smoked paprika.

Kibbeh

PREP TIME: 10 MINUTES / COOK TIME: 20 MINUTES/ SERVES 2

Ingredients
1 cup medium-grind bulgur, rinsed
1 cup water
8 ounces ground lamb
1 small onion, chopped
½ teaspoon ground cinnamon
½ teaspoon salt
¼ teaspoon pepper
1 teaspoon extra-virgin olive oil
8 ounces ground lamb

Salt and pepper
1 small onion, chopped fine
½ cup pine nuts, toasted
½ teaspoon ground cinnamon
⅛ teaspoon ground allspice
1 tablespoon pomegranate molasses
2 cups vegetable oil

Directions
Preparing the Ingredients
1. For the dough: Combine bulgur and water in bowl and let sit until grains begin to soften, 30 to 40 minutes. Drain bulgur well and transfer to bowl of food processor. Add lamb, onion, cinnamon, salt, and pepper and process to smooth paste, about 1 minute, scraping down sides of bowl as needed. Transfer dough to bowl, cover, and refrigerate until chilled, about 30 minutes.
2. For the filling: Heat oil in 12-inch skillet over medium-high heat until just smoking. Add lamb, ½ teaspoon salt, and ¼ teaspoon pepper and cook, breaking up meat with wooden spoon, until browned, 3 to 5 minutes. Using slotted spoon, transfer meat to paper towel–lined plate. Pour off all but 1 tablespoon fat from skillet.
3. Add onion to fat left in skillet and cook over medium heat until softened, about 5 minutes. Stir in pine nuts, cinnamon, and allspice and cook until fragrant, about 30 seconds. Off heat, stir in lamb and pomegranate molasses and season with salt and pepper to taste.
4. Line rimmed baking sheet with parchment paper and grease parchment. Pinch off and roll dough into 2-inch balls (16 balls total). Working with 1 dough ball at a time, use your lightly oiled hands to press and stretch dough into rough cup with ¼-inch-thick sides. Spoon 1 tablespoon filling into cup, pressing gently to pack filling, and pinch seam closed. Gently form kibbeh into 3 by 1½-inch torpedo shape with tapered ends and transfer to prepared sheet. Cover and refrigerate kibbeh until firm, at least 30 minutes or up to 24 hours.
5. Adjust oven rack to middle position and heat oven to 200 degrees. Set wire rack in second rimmed baking sheet and line with triple layer of paper towels. Heat oil in clean 12-inch skillet over medium-high heat to 375 degrees.
6. Fry half of kibbeh until deep golden brown, 2 to 3 minutes per side. Adjust burner, if necessary, to maintain oil temperature of 375 degrees. Using slotted spoon, transfer kibbeh to prepared rack and keep warm in oven. Return oil to 375 degrees and repeat with remaining kibbeh.

Braised Short Ribs with Fennel and Pickled Grapes

PREP TIME: 10 MINUTES / COOK TIME: 20 MINUTES/ SERVES 4

Ingredients

1½ pounds boneless beef short ribs, trimmed and cut into 2-inch pieces
1 teaspoon table salt, divided
1 tablespoon extra-virgin olive oil
1 fennel bulb, 2 tablespoons fronds chopped, stalks discarded, bulb halved, cored, and sliced into 1-inch-thick wedges
1 onion, halved and sliced ½ inch thick
4 garlic cloves, minced
2 teaspoons fennel seeds
½ cup chicken broth
1 sprig fresh rosemary
¼ cup red wine vinegar
1 tablespoon sugar
4 ounces seedless red grapes, halved (½ cup)

Directions

1. Pat short ribs dry with paper towels and sprinkle with ½ teaspoon salt. Using highest sauté function, heat oil in Instant Pot for 5 minutes (or until just smoking). Brown short ribs on all sides, 6 to 8 minutes; transfer to plate.

2. Add fennel wedges, onion, and ¼ teaspoon salt to fat left in pot and cook, using highest sauté function, until vegetables are softened and lightly browned, about 5 minutes. Stir in garlic and fennel seeds and cook until fragrant, about 30 seconds. Stir in broth and rosemary sprig, scraping up any browned bits. Nestle short ribs into vegetable mixture and add any accumulated juices. Lock lid in place and close pressure release valve. Select high pressure cook function and cook for 35 minutes.

3. Meanwhile, microwave vinegar, sugar, and remaining ¼ teaspoon salt in bowl until simmering, about 1 minute. Add grapes and let sit, stirring occasionally, for 20 minutes. Drain grapes and return to now-empty bowl. (Drained grapes can be refrigerated for up to 1 week.)

4. Turn off Instant Pot and let pressure release naturally for 15 minutes. Quick-release any remaining pressure, then carefully remove lid, allowing steam to escape away from you. Transfer short ribs to serving dish, tent with aluminum foil, and let rest while finishing sauce.

5. Strain braising liquid through fine-mesh strainer into fat separator. Discard rosemary sprig and transfer vegetables to serving dish with beef. Let braising liquid settle for 5 minutes, then pour ¾ cup defatted liquid over short ribs and vegetables; discard remaining liquid. Sprinkle with grapes and fennel fronds. Serve.

Moroccan Meatballs

PREP TIME: 10 MINUTES / COOK TIME: 20 MINUTES/ SERVES 4

Ingredients

¼ cup finely chopped onion (about ⅛ onion)
¼ cup raisins, coarsely chopped
1 teaspoon ground cumin
½ teaspoon ground cinnamon
¼ teaspoon smoked paprika
1 large egg
1 pound ground beef (93% lean) or ground lamb
⅓ cup panko bread crumbs
1 teaspoon extra-virgin olive oil
1 (28-ounce) can low-sodium or no-salt-added crushed tomatoes
Chopped fresh mint, feta cheese, and/or fresh orange or lemon wedges, for serving (optional)

Directions

1. **Preparing the Ingredients**
In a large bowl, combine the onion, raisins, cumin, cinnamon, smoked paprika, and egg. Add the ground beef and bread crumbs and mix gently with your hands. Divide the mixture into 20 even portions, then wet your hands and roll each portion into a ball. Wash your hands.

2. **Cooking**
In a large skillet over medium-high heat, heat the oil. Add the meatballs and cook for 8 minutes, rolling around every minute or so with tongs or a fork to brown them on most sides. (They won't be cooked through.) Transfer the meatballs to a paper towel–lined plate. Drain the fat out of the pan, and carefully wipe out the hot pan with a paper towel.
Return the meatballs to the pan, and pour the tomatoes over the meatballs. Cover and cook on medium-high heat until the sauce begins to bubble. Lower the heat to medium, cover partially, and cook for 7 to 8 more minutes, until the meatballs are cooked through. Garnish with fresh mint, feta cheese, and/or a squeeze of citrus, if desired, and serve.

Beef Kofta

PREP TIME: 10 MINUTES / COOK TIME: 20 MINUTES/ SERVES 4

Ingredients

Olive oil cooking spray
½ onion, roughly chopped
1-inch piece ginger, peeled
2 garlic cloves, peeled
⅓ cup fresh parsley
⅓ cup fresh mint
1 pound ground beef
1 tablespoon ground cumin
1 tablespoon ground coriander
1 teaspoon ground cinnamon
¾ teaspoon kosher salt
½ teaspoon ground sumac
¼ teaspoon ground cloves
¼ teaspoon freshly ground black pepper

Directions

1. **Preparing the Ingredients**
Preheat the oven to 400°F. Grease a 12-cup muffin tin with olive oil cooking spray.
In a food processor, add the onion, ginger, garlic, parsley, and mint; process until minced.
Place the onion mixture in a large bowl. Add the beef, cumin, coriander, cinnamon, salt, sumac, cloves, and black pepper and mix together thoroughly with your

hands. Divide the beef mixture into 12 balls and place each one in a cup of the prepared muffin tin.

2.   Cooking

Bake for 20 minutes. Ground lamb, turkey, chicken, and pork should all work well here. If using meat with less fat, such as poultry breast or pork, the cooking time may decrease by 2 to 3 minutes so that the kofta does not dry out.

Dijon and Herb Pork Tenderloin

PREP TIME: 10 MINUTES / COOK TIME: 20 MINUTES (PLUS 10 MINUTES TO REST) / SERVES 6

Ingredients

½ cup fresh Italian parsley leaves, chopped
3 tablespoons fresh rosemary leaves, chopped
3 tablespoons fresh thyme leaves, chopped
3 tablespoons Dijon mustard
1 tablespoon extra-virgin olive oil
4 garlic cloves, minced
½ teaspoon sea salt
¼ teaspoon freshly ground black pepper
1 (1½-pound) pork tenderloin

Directions

1.   Preparing the Ingredients

Preheat the oven to 400°F. In a blender or food processor, combine the parsley, rosemary, thyme, mustard, olive oil, garlic, sea salt, and pepper. Process for about 30 seconds until smooth.
Spread the mixture evenly over the pork and place it on a rimmed baking sheet.

2.   Cooking

Bake for about 20 minutes, or until the meat reaches an internal temperature of 140°F. Remove from the oven and let rest for 10 minutes before slicing and serving.

Wine-Braised Short Ribs with Potatoes (Instant Pot)

PREP TIME: 15 MINUTES / COOK TIME: 1 HOUR / SERVES 4

Ingredients

2 pounds bone-in English-style beef short ribs, trimmed
¾ teaspoon table salt, divided
¼ teaspoon pepper
1 tablespoon extra-virgin olive oil
1 onion, chopped fine
6 garlic cloves, minced
2 tablespoons tomato paste
1 tablespoon minced fresh oregano or 1 teaspoon dried
1 (14.5-ounce) can whole peeled tomatoes, drained with ¼ cup juice reserved, chopped coarse
½ cup dry red wine
1 pound small red potatoes, unpeeled, halved
2 tablespoons minced fresh parsley

Directions

1.   Pat short ribs dry with paper towels and sprinkle with ½ teaspoon salt and pepper. Using

highest sauté function, heat oil in Instant Pot for 5 minutes (or until just smoking). Brown short ribs on all sides, 6 to 8 minutes; transfer to plate.

2.   Add onion and remaining ¼ teaspoon salt to fat left in pot and cook, using highest sauté function, until onion is softened, about 3 minutes. Stir in garlic, tomato paste, and oregano and cook until fragrant, about 30 seconds. Stir in tomatoes and reserved juice and wine, scraping up any browned bits. Nestle short ribs meat side down into pot and add any accumulated juices. Lock lid in place and close pressure release valve. Select high pressure cook function and cook for 60 minutes.

3.   Turn off Instant Pot and let pressure release naturally for 15 minutes. Quick-release any remaining pressure, then carefully remove lid, allowing steam to escape away from you. Transfer short ribs to serving dish, tent with aluminum foil, and let rest while preparing potatoes.

4.   Strain braising liquid through fine-mesh strainer into fat separator; transfer solids to now-empty pot. Let braising liquid settle for 5 minutes, then pour 1½ cups defatted liquid and any accumulated juices into pot with solids; discard remaining liquid. Add potatoes. Lock lid in place and close pressure release valve. Select high pressure cook function and cook for 4 minutes. Turn off Instant Pot and quick-release pressure. Carefully remove lid, allowing steam to escape away from you.

5.   Using slotted spoon, transfer potatoes to serving dish. Season sauce with salt and pepper to taste. Spoon sauce over short ribs and potatoes and sprinkle with parsley. Serve.

Beef Spanakopita Pita Pockets

PREP TIME: 5 MINUTES / COOK TIME: 15 MINUTES / SERVES 4

Ingredients

3 teaspoons extra-virgin olive oil, divided
1 pound ground beef (93% lean)
2 garlic cloves, minced (about 1 teaspoon)
2 (6-ounce) bags baby spinach, chopped (about 12 cups)
½ cup crumbled feta cheese (about 2 ounces)
⅓ cup ricotta cheese
½ teaspoon ground nutmeg
¼ teaspoon freshly ground black pepper
¼ cup slivered almonds
4 (6-inch) whole-wheat pita breads, cut in half

Directions

Preparing the Ingredients

1.   In a large skillet over medium heat, heat 1 teaspoon of oil. Add the ground beef and cook for 10 minutes, breaking it up with a wooden spoon and stirring occasionally. Remove from the heat and drain in a colander. Set the meat aside.

2.   Place the skillet back on the heat, and add the remaining 2 teaspoons of oil. Add the garlic and cook for 1 minute, stirring constantly. Add the

spinach and cook for 2 to 3 minutes, or until the spinach has cooked down, stirring often.

3. Turn off the heat and mix in the feta cheese, ricotta, nutmeg, and pepper. Stir until all the ingredients are well incorporated. Mix in the almonds.

Divide the beef filling among the eight pita pocket halves to stuff them and serve.

Mediterranean Chimichurri Skirt Steak

PREP TIME: 10 MINUTES, PLUS 30 MINUTES TO MARINATE / COOK TIME: 15 MINUTES / SERVES 4

Ingredients

¾ cup fresh mint
¾ cup fresh parsley
⅔ cup extra-virgin olive oil
⅓ cup lemon juice
Zest of 1 lemon
2 tablespoons dried oregano
4 garlic cloves, peeled
½ teaspoon red pepper flakes
½ teaspoon kosher salt
1 to 1½ pounds skirt steak, cut in half if longer than grill pan

Directions

1. Preparing the Ingredients

In a food processor or blender, add the mint, parsley, olive oil, lemon juice, lemon zest, oregano, garlic, red pepper flakes, and salt. Process until the mixture reaches your desired consistency—anywhere from a slightly chunky to smooth purée. Remove a half cup of the chimichurri mixture and set aside.

Pour the remaining chimichurri mixture into a medium bowl or zip-top bag and add the steak. Mix together well and marinate for at least 30 minutes, and up to 8 hours in the refrigerator.

2. Cooking

In a grill pan over medium-high heat, add the steak and cook 4 minutes on each side (for medium rare). Cook an additional 1 to 2 minutes per side for medium.

Place the steak on a cutting board, tent with foil to keep it warm, and let it rest for 10 minutes. Thinly slice the steak crosswise against the grain and serve with the reserved sauce.

Prep the chimichurri sauce the day before, then in the morning place the steak and sauce in a zip-top bag, put it in the refrigerator, and go about your day. When it's dinnertime, you'll have the steak ready to go and cooked in less than 15 minutes.

Steak With Red Wine–Mushroom Sauce

PREP TIME: 10 MINUTES (PLUS 4 TO 8 HOURS TO MARINATE) / COOK TIME: 20 MINUTES / SERVES 4

Ingredients

1 cup dry red wine
3 garlic cloves, minced
2 tablespoons extra-virgin olive oil
1 tablespoon low-sodium soy sauce
1 tablespoon dried thyme
1 teaspoon Dijon mustard
2 tablespoons extra-virgin olive oil
1 to 1½ pounds skirt steak, flat iron steak, or tri-tip steak
2 tablespoons extra-virgin olive oil
1 pound cremini mushrooms, quartered
½ teaspoon sea salt
1 teaspoon dried thyme
⅛ teaspoon freshly ground black pepper
2 garlic cloves, minced
1 cup dry red wine

Directions

Preparing the Ingredients

1. To make the marinade and steak

In a small bowl, whisk the wine, garlic, olive oil, soy sauce, thyme, and mustard. Pour into a resealable bag and add the steak. Refrigerate the steak to marinate for 4 to 8 hours. Remove the steak from the marinade and pat it dry with paper towels.

In a large skillet over medium-high heat, heat the olive oil until it shimmers.

Add the steak and cook for about 4 minutes per side until deeply browned on each side and the steak reaches an internal temperature of 140°F. Remove the steak from the skillet and put it on a plate tented with aluminum foil to keep warm, while you prepare the mushroom sauce.

When the mushroom sauce is ready, slice the steak against the grain into ½-inch-thick slices.

2. In the same skillet over medium-high heat, heat the olive oil until it shimmers.

Add the mushrooms, sea salt, thyme, and pepper. Cook for about 6 minutes, stirring very infrequently, until the mushrooms are browned.

Add the garlic and cook for 30 seconds, stirring constantly.

Stir in the wine, and use the side of a wooden spoon to scrape and fold in any browned bits from the bottom of the skillet. Cook for about 4 minutes, stirring occasionally, until the liquid reduces by half. Serve the mushrooms spooned over the steak.

3. The trick to cooking really tasty mushrooms is to leave them alone as much as possible. Let the mushrooms sit in contact with the pan for at least 2 minutes before you stir them. Stir only 2 or 3 times during the cooking process to promote browning and prevent burning. You'll know they are ready when they have released their liquid and it has evaporated, and the mushrooms are well browned on all sides.

Greek-Style Ground Beef Pita Sandwiches

PREP TIME: 15 MINUTES / COOK TIME: 0 MINUTES / SERVES 2

Ingredients

1 tablespoon olive oil
½ medium onion, minced
2 garlic cloves, minced
6 ounces lean ground beef
1 teaspoon dried oregano

For the yogurt sauce

⅓ cup plain Greek yogurt

1 ounce crumbled feta cheese (about 3 tablespoons)

1 tablespoon minced fresh parsley

1 tablespoon minced scallion

1 tablespoon freshly squeezed lemon juice

Pinch salt

For the sandwiches

2 large Greek-style pitas

½ cup cherry tomatoes, halved

1 cup diced cucumber

Salt

Freshly ground black pepper

Directions

Preparing the Ingredients

1.   Warm the pitas in the microwave for 20 seconds each.

2.   To serve, spread some of the yogurt sauce over each warm pita. Top with the ground beef, cherry tomatoes, and diced cucumber. Season with salt and pepper. Add additional yogurt sauce if desired.

If you prefer, you can make these with ground chicken or turkey breast instead of beef.

Grilled Steak, Mushroom, and Onion Kebabs

PREP TIME: 10 MINUTES / COOK TIME: 10 MINUTES / SERVES 4

Ingredients

Nonstick cooking spray

4 garlic cloves, peeled

2 fresh rosemary sprigs (about 3 inches each)

2 tablespoons extra-virgin olive oil, divided

1 pound boneless top sirloin steak, about 1 inch thick

1 (8-ounce) package white button mushrooms

1 medium red onion, cut into 12 thin wedges

¼ teaspoon coarsely ground black pepper

2 tablespoons red wine vinegar

¼ teaspoon kosher or sea salt

Directions

Preparing the Ingredients

1.   Soak 12 (10-inch) wooden skewers in water. Spray the cold grill with nonstick cooking spray, and heat the grill to medium-high.

2.   Cut a piece of aluminum foil into a 10-inch square. Place the garlic and rosemary sprigs in the center, drizzle with 1 tablespoon of oil, and wrap tightly to form a foil packet. Place it on the grill, and close the grill cover.

3.   Cut the steak into 1-inch cubes. Thread the beef onto the wet skewers, alternating with whole mushrooms and onion wedges. Spray the kebabs thoroughly with nonstick cooking spray, and sprinkle with pepper.

4.   Cook the kebabs on the covered grill for 4 to 5 minutes. Turn and grill 4 to 5 more minutes, covered, until a meat thermometer inserted in the meat registers 145°F (medium rare) or 160°F (medium).

5.   Remove the foil packet from the grill, open, and, using tongs, place the garlic and rosemary sprigs in a small bowl. Carefully strip the rosemary sprigs of their leaves into the bowl and pour in any accumulated juices and oil from the foil packet. Add the remaining 1 tablespoon of oil and the vinegar and salt. Mash the garlic with a fork, and mix all ingredients in the bowl together. Pour over the finished steak kebabs and serve.

Lamb Meatballs

PREP TIME: 10 MINUTES / COOK TIME: 20 MINUTES / SERVES 4

Ingredients

Olive oil cooking spray

1 pound ground lamb

¼ cup fresh mint, chopped

¼ cup shallot, chopped

1 large egg, beaten

1 garlic clove, chopped

1 teaspoon ground coriander

1 teaspoon ground cumin

½ teaspoon kosher salt

¼ teaspoon ground cinnamon

¼ teaspoon red pepper flakes

Directions

1.   **Preparing the Ingredients**

Preheat the oven to 400°F. Grease a 12-cup muffin tin with olive oil cooking spray.

In a large bowl, combine the lamb, mint, shallot, egg, garlic, coriander, cumin, salt, cinnamon, and red pepper flakes; mix well. Form the mixture into 12 balls and place one in each cup of the prepared muffin tin.

2.   **Cooking**

Bake for 20 minutes, or until golden brown. A single portion of lamb provides a variety of essential vitamins and minerals, including iron, vitamin B12, niacin, zinc, selenium, and omega-3 fatty acids. Lean lamb is a source of healthy, unsaturated fats, with nearly 40 percent coming from monounsaturated fat. Ground beef or poultry can be used in place of the lamb, if preferred.

Greek Meatballs

PREP TIME: 20 MINUTES / COOK TIME: 25 MINUTES / SERVES 4

Ingredients

2 whole-wheat bread slices

1¼ pounds ground turkey

1 egg

¼ cup seasoned whole-wheat bread crumbs

3 garlic cloves, minced

¼ red onion, grated

¼ cup chopped fresh Italian parsley leaves

2 tablespoons chopped fresh mint leaves

2 tablespoons chopped fresh oregano leaves

½ teaspoon sea salt

¼ teaspoon freshly ground black pepper

Directions

1. **Preparing the Ingredients**

Preheat the oven to 350°F. Line a baking sheet with parchment paper or aluminum foil.

2. Run the bread under water to wet it, and squeeze out any excess. Tear the wet bread into small pieces and place it in a medium bowl. Add the turkey, egg, bread crumbs, garlic, red onion, parsley, mint, oregano, sea salt, and pepper. Mix well. Form the mixture into ¼-cup-size balls. Place the meatballs on the prepared sheet and bake for about 25 minutes, or until the internal temperature reaches 165°F.

Lemon Herb-Crusted Pork Tenderloin

PREP TIME: 10 MINUTES / COOK TIME: 20 MINUTES / SERVES 2

Ingredients

1 (8-ounce) pork tenderloin
Zest of 1 lemon
½ teaspoon dried thyme
¼ teaspoon garlic powder
¼ teaspoon za'atar seasoning
¼ teaspoon salt
1 tablespoon olive oil

Directions

1. **Preparing the Ingredients**

Preheat the oven to 425°F and set the rack to the middle position.

Trim away any of the silver skin from the pork tenderloin, to prevent it from curling while it cooks. Combine the lemon zest, thyme, garlic powder, za'atar, and salt in a small bowl. Rub it evenly over the pork tenderloin.

2. **Cooking**.

Heat the olive oil in a sauté pan over medium-high heat. Add the pork and sauté for 3 minutes, turning often, until it's golden on all sides.

Place the tenderloin in an oven-safe baking dish and roast for 15 minutes, or until the internal temperature registers 145°F. Remove it from the oven and let it rest for 3 minutes before serving.

Grilled Flank Steak With Grilled Vegetables And Salsa Verde

PREP TIME: 5 MINUTES / COOK TIME: 15 MINUTES / SERVES 4 TO 6

Ingredients

1 red onion, sliced into ½-inch-thick rounds
8 ounces cherry tomatoes
2 zucchini, sliced lengthwise into ¾-inch-thick planks
1 pound eggplant, sliced lengthwise into ¾-inch-thick planks
2 tablespoons extra-virgin olive oil
1½ pounds flank steak, trimmed
Salt and pepper
½ cup Italian Salsa Verde

Directions

Preparing the Ingredients.

Thread onion rounds from side to side onto two 12-inch metal skewers. Thread cherry tomatoes onto two 12-inch metal skewers. Brush onion rounds, tomatoes, zucchini, and eggplant with oil and season with salt and pepper.

Pat steak dry with paper towels and season with salt and pepper.

For a charcoal grill: Open bottom grill vent completely.

Light large chimney starter filled with charcoal briquettes (6 quarts). When top coals are partially covered with ash, pour evenly over grill. Set cooking grate in place, cover, and open lid vent completely. Heat grill until hot, about 5 minutes.

For a gas grill grill: Turn all burners to high, cover, and heat grill until hot, about 15 minutes. Leave all burners on high.

Clean and oil cooking grate. Place steak, onion and tomato skewers, zucchini, and eggplant on grill. Cook (covered if using gas), flipping steak and turning vegetables as needed, until steak is well browned and registers 120 to 125 degrees (for medium-rare) and vegetables are slightly charred and tender, 7 to 12 minutes.

Transfer steak and vegetables to carving board as they finish grilling and tent loosely with aluminum foil. Let steak rest for 10 minutes.

Meanwhile, slide tomatoes and onions off skewers using tongs.

Cut onion rounds, zucchini, and eggplant into 2- to 3-inch pieces. Arrange vegetables on serving platter and season with salt and pepper to taste. Slice steak thin against grain on bias and arrange on platter with vegetables.

Drizzle steak with ¼ cup Salsa Verde. Serve, passing remaining sauce separately.

Italian Salsa Verde

PREP TIME: 5 MINUTES / COOK TIME: NONE / MAKE 1 CUO / SERVES 4

Ingredients

3 cups fresh parsley leaves
1 cup fresh mint leaves
½ cup extra-virgin olive oil
3 tablespoons white wine vinegar
2 tablespoons capers, rinsed
3 anchovy fillets, rinsed
1 garlic clove, minced
⅛ teaspoon salt

Directions

Preparing the Ingredients

Pulse all ingredients in food processor until mixture is finely chopped (mixture should not be smooth), about 10 pulses, scraping down sides of bowl as needed. Transfer mixture to bowl and serve. (Sauce can be refrigerated for up to 2 days; bring to room temperature before serving.

Beef Gyros with Tahini Sauce

PREP TIME: 10 MINUTES / COOK TIME: 15 MINUTES / SERVES 4

Ingredients

Nonstick cooking spray

2 tablespoons extra-virgin olive oil
1 tablespoon dried oregano
1¼ teaspoons garlic powder, divided
1 teaspoon ground cumin
½ teaspoon freshly ground black pepper
¼ teaspoon kosher or sea salt
1 pound beef flank steak, top round steak, or lamb leg steak, center cut, about 1 inch thick
1 medium green bell pepper, halved and seeded
2 tablespoons tahini or peanut butter (tahini for nut-free)
1 tablespoon hot water (if needed)
½ cup 2% plain Greek yogurt
1 tablespoon freshly squeezed lemon juice (about ½ small lemon)
1 cup thinly sliced red onion (about ½ onion)
4 (6-inch) whole-wheat pita breads, warmed

Directions

1.   Preparing the Ingredients
Set an oven rack about 4 inches below the broiler element. Preheat the oven broiler to high. Line a large, rimmed baking sheet with foil. Place a wire cooling rack on the foil, and spray the rack with nonstick cooking spray. Set aside.

In a small bowl, whisk together the oil, oregano, 1 teaspoon of garlic powder, cumin, pepper, and salt. Rub the oil mixture on all sides of the steak, saving 1 teaspoon of the mixture. Place the steak on the prepared rack. Rub the remaining oil mixture on the bell pepper, and place on the rack, cut-side down. Press the pepper with the heel of your hand to flatten.

2.   Cooking.
Broil for 5 minutes. Turn the meat and the pepper pieces, and broil for 2 to 5 more minutes, until the pepper is charred and the internal temperature of the meat measures 145°F on a meat thermometer. Put the pepper and steak on a cutting board to rest for 5 minutes.

While the meat is broiling, in a small bowl, whisk the tahini until smooth (adding 1 tablespoon of hot water if your tahini is sticky). Add the remaining ¼ teaspoon of garlic powder and the yogurt and lemon juice, and whisk thoroughly.

Slice the steak crosswise into ¼-inch-thick strips. Slice the bell pepper into strips. Divide the steak, bell pepper, and onion among the warm pita breads. Drizzle with tahini sauce and serve.

Ground Lamb with Lentils and Pomegranate Seeds

PREP TIME: 15 MINUTES / COOK TIME: 15 MINUTES / SERVES 4

Ingredients

1 tablespoon extra-virgin olive oil
½ pound ground lamb
1 teaspoon red pepper flakes
½ teaspoon ground cumin
½ teaspoon kosher salt
¼ teaspoon freshly ground black pepper
2 garlic cloves, minced
2 cups cooked, drained lentils
1 hothouse or English cucumber, diced
⅓ cup fresh mint, chopped
⅓ cup fresh parsley, chopped
Zest of 1 lemon
1 cup plain Greek yogurt
½ cup pomegranate seeds

Directions

Preparing the Ingredients

1.   Heat the olive oil in a large skillet or sauté pan over medium-high heat. Add the lamb and season with the red pepper flakes, cumin, salt, and black pepper. Cook the lamb without stirring until the bottom is brown and crispy, about 5 minutes. Stir and cook for another 5 minutes. Using a spatula, break up the lamb into smaller pieces. Add the garlic and cook, stirring occasionally, for 1 minute. Transfer the lamb mixture to a medium bowl.

2.   Add the lentils to the skillet and cook, stirring occasionally, until brown and crisp, about 5 minutes. Return the lamb to the skillet, mix, and warm through, about 3 minutes. Transfer to the large bowl. Add the cucumber, mint, parsley, and lemon zest, mixing together gently. Spoon the yogurt into 4 bowls and top each with some of the lamb mixture. Garnish with the pomegranate seeds.

RICE AND BEANS

Spiced Rice Pilaf with Sweet Potatoes and Pomegranate (Instant Pot)

PREP TIME: 22 MINUTES / COOK TIME: 23 MINUTES/ SERVES 4 TO 6

Ingredients

2 tablespoons extra-virgin olive oil
1 onion, chopped fine
½ teaspoon table salt
2 garlic cloves, minced
1½ teaspoons ground turmeric
1 teaspoon ground coriander
⅛ teaspoon cayenne pepper
2 cups chicken broth
1½ cups long-grain white rice, rinsed
12 ounces sweet potato, peeled, quartered lengthwise, and sliced ½ inch thick
½ preserved lemon, pulp and white pith removed, rind rinsed and minced (2 tablespoons)
½ cup shelled pistachios, toasted and chopped
¼ cup fresh cilantro leaves
¼ cup pomegranate seeds

Directions

1.   Using highest sauté function, heat oil in Instant Pot until shimmering. Add onion and salt and cook until onion is softened, about 5 minutes. Stir in garlic, turmeric, coriander, and cayenne and cook until fragrant, about 30 seconds. Stir in broth, rice, and sweet potato.

2.   Lock lid in place and close pressure release valve. Select high pressure cook function and cook for 4 minutes. Turn off Instant Pot and quick-release pressure. Carefully remove lid, allowing steam to escape away from you.

3.   Add preserved lemon and gently fluff rice with fork to combine. Lay clean dish towel over pot, replace lid, and let sit for 5 minutes. Season with salt and pepper to taste. Transfer to serving dish and sprinkle with pistachios, cilantro, and pomegranate seeds. Serve.

Italian Baked Beans

PREP TIME: 5 MINUTES / COOK TIME: 15 MINUTES/ SERVES 6

Ingredients

2 teaspoons extra-virgin olive oil
½ cup minced onion (about ¼ onion)
1 (12-ounce) can low-sodium tomato paste
¼ cup red wine vinegar
2 tablespoons honey
¼ teaspoon ground cinnamon
½ cup water
2 (15-ounce) cans cannellini or great northern beans, undrained

Directions

Preparing the Ingredients

1.   In a medium saucepan over medium heat, heat the oil. Add the onion and cook for 5 minutes, stirring frequently. Add the tomato paste, vinegar, honey, cinnamon, and water, and mix well. Turn the heat to low.

2.   Drain and rinse one can of the beans in a colander and add to the saucepan. Pour the entire second can of beans (including the liquid) into the saucepan. Let it cook for 10 minutes, stirring occasionally, and serve.

Farro with Artichoke Hearts

PREP TIME: 10 MINUTES / COOK TIME: 40 MINUTES/ SERVES 6

Ingredients

1 cup farro
1 bay leaf
1 fresh rosemary sprig
1 fresh thyme sprig
2 tablespoons extra-virgin olive oil
1 onion, chopped
2 cups frozen artichoke hearts, thawed and chopped
1 tablespoon Italian seasoning
3 garlic cloves, minced
2 cups unsalted vegetable broth
Zest of 1 lemon
½ teaspoon sea salt
⅛ teaspoon freshly ground black pepper
¼ cup (about 2 ounces) grated Parmesan cheese

Directions

1.   **Preparing the Ingredients**. In a medium pot, combine the farro, bay leaf, rosemary, and thyme with enough water to cover it by about 2 inches.

2.   **Cooking**. Place it on the stove top over medium-high heat and bring it to a boil. Reduce the heat to medium-low and simmer uncovered for 25 to 30 minutes, stirring occasionally, until the grain is tender. Drain any excess water and set the farro aside. Remove and discard the bay leaf, rosemary, and thyme. In a large skillet over medium-high heat, heat the olive oil until it shimmers. Add the onion, artichoke hearts, and Italian seasoning. Cook for about 5 minutes, stirring frequently, until the onion is soft. Add the garlic and cook for 30 seconds, stirring constantly. Add the broth, ½ cup at a time, and stir constantly until the liquid is absorbed before adding the next ½ cup of broth. Stir in the lemon zest, sea salt, pepper, and cheese. Cook for 1 to 2 minutes more, stirring, until the cheese melts.

Replace the farro with 2 cups cooked brown rice and reduce the broth to 1 cup.

Cannellini Bean Lettuce Wraps

PREP TIME: 10 MINUTES / COOK TIME: 10 MINUTES/ SERVES 4

Ingredients

1 tablespoon extra-virgin olive oil
½ cup diced red onion (about ¼ onion)
¾ cup chopped fresh tomatoes (about 1 medium tomato)

¼ teaspoon freshly ground black pepper
1 (15-ounce) can cannellini or great northern beans, drained and rinsed
¼ cup finely chopped fresh curly parsley
½ cup Lemony Garlic Hummus or ½ cup prepared hummus
8 romaine lettuce leaves

Directions
Preparing the Ingredients

1.	In a large skillet over medium heat, heat the oil. Add the onion and cook for 3 minutes, stirring occasionally. Add the tomatoes and pepper and cook for 3 more minutes, stirring occasionally. Add the beans and cook for 3 more minutes, stirring occasionally. Remove from the heat, and mix in the parsley.

2.	Spread 1 tablespoon of hummus over each lettuce leaf. Evenly spread the warm bean mixture down the center of each leaf. Fold one side of the lettuce leaf over the filling lengthwise, then fold over the other side to make a wrap and serve.

Rice and Spinach

PREP TIME: 10 MINUTES / COOK TIME: 15 MINUTES/ SERVES 6

Ingredients
2 tablespoons extra-virgin olive oil
1 onion, chopped
4 cups fresh baby spinach
1 garlic clove, minced
Zest of 1 orange
Juice of 1 orange
1 cup unsalted vegetable broth
½ teaspoon sea salt
⅛ teaspoon freshly ground black pepper
2 cups cooked brown rice

Directions
Preparing the Ingredients

1.	In a large skillet over medium-high heat, heat the olive oil until it shimmers. Add the onion and cook for about 5 minutes, stirring occasionally, until soft. Add the spinach and cook for about 2 minutes, stirring occasionally, until it wilts. Add the garlic and cook for 30 seconds, stirring constantly. Stir in the orange zest and juice, broth, sea salt, and pepper. Bring to a simmer. Stir in the rice and cook for about 4 minutes, stirring, until the rice is heated through and the liquid is absorbed.

2.	Save time by cooking the rice ahead of time and freezing it in handy 1-cup servings for up to 6 months. 8 If you plan to freeze this dish, it's best to use freshly cooked rice, not frozen.

Spiced Couscous

PREP TIME: 10 MINUTES / COOK TIME: 15 MINUTES/ SERVES 6

Ingredients
2 tablespoons extra-virgin olive oil
½ onion, minced
Juice of 1 orange

Zest of 1 orange
½ teaspoon garlic powder
½ teaspoon ground cumin
½ teaspoon sea salt
¼ teaspoon ground ginger
¼ teaspoon ground allspice
¼ teaspoon ground cinnamon
⅛ teaspoon freshly ground black pepper
2 cups water
1 cup whole-wheat couscous
¼ cup dried apricots, chopped
¼ cup dried cranberries

Directions
Preparing the Ingredients

1.	In a medium saucepan over medium-high heat, heat the olive oil until it shimmers. Add the onion and cook for about 3 minutes, stirring occasionally, until soft. Add the orange juice and zest, garlic powder, cumin, sea salt, ginger, allspice, cinnamon, pepper, and water. Bring to a boil. Add the couscous, apricots, and cranberries. Stir once, turn off the heat, and cover the pot. Let rest for 5 minutes, covered. Fluff with a fork.
Add ¼ cup pine nuts in place of the dried apricots for a little crunch.

2.	Couscous freezes well for up to 6 months, so you can save it in ¾-cup serving sizes in resealable bags or tightly sealed containers for a quick side dish.

Bulgur with Chickpeas, Spinach, and Za'atar (Instant Pot)

PREP TIME: 22 MINUTES / COOK TIME: 1 MINUTE/ SERVES 4 TO 6

Ingredients
3 tablespoons extra-virgin olive oil, divided
1 onion, chopped fine
½ teaspoon table salt
3 garlic cloves, minced
2 tablespoons za'atar, divided
1 cup medium-grind bulgur, rinsed
1 (15-ounce) can chickpeas, rinsed
1½ cups water
5 ounces (5 cups) baby spinach, chopped
1 tablespoon lemon juice, plus lemon wedges for serving

Directions

1.	Using highest sauté function, heat 2 tablespoons oil in Instant Pot until shimmering. Add onion and salt and cook until onion is softened, about 5 minutes. Stir in garlic and 1 tablespoon za'atar and cook until fragrant, about 30 seconds. Stir in bulgur, chickpeas, and water.

2.	Lock lid in place and close pressure release valve. Select high pressure cook function and cook for 1 minute. Turn off Instant Pot and quick-release pressure. Carefully remove lid, allowing steam to escape away from you.

3.	Gently fluff bulgur with fork. Lay clean dish towel over pot, replace lid, and let sit for 5 minutes. Add spinach, lemon juice, remaining 1 tablespoon za'atar, and remaining 1 tablespoon oil and gently toss to combine. Season with salt and pepper to taste. Serve with lemon wedges.

Mediterranean Lentils and Rice

PREP TIME: 10 MINUTES / COOK TIME: 20 MINUTES/ SERVES 4

Ingredients

2¼ cups low-sodium or no-salt-added vegetable broth
½ cup uncooked brown or green lentils
½ cup uncooked instant brown rice
½ cup diced carrots (about 1 carrot)
½ cup diced celery (about 1 stalk)
1 (2.25-ounce) can sliced olives, drained (about ½ cup)
¼ cup diced red onion (about ⅛ onion)
¼ cup chopped fresh curly-leaf parsley
1½ tablespoons extra-virgin olive oil
1 tablespoon freshly squeezed lemon juice (from about ½ small lemon)
1 garlic clove, minced (about ½ teaspoon)
¼ teaspoon kosher or sea salt
¼ teaspoon freshly ground black pepper

Directions

Preparing the Ingredients

1.   In a medium saucepan over high heat, bring the broth and lentils to a boil, cover, and lower the heat to medium-low. Cook for 8 minutes.
2.   Raise the heat to medium, and stir in the rice. Cover the pot and cook the mixture for 15 minutes, or until the liquid is absorbed. Remove the pot from the heat and let it sit, covered, for 1 minute, then stir.
3.   While the lentils and rice are cooking, mix together the carrots, celery, olives, onion, and parsley in a large serving bowl.
4.   In a small bowl, whisk together the oil, lemon juice, garlic, salt, and pepper. Set aside. When the lentils and rice are cooked, add them to the serving bowl. Pour the dressing on top, and mix everything together. Serve warm or cold, or store in a sealed container in the refrigerator for up to 7 days.

Sweet Potato Mash

PREP TIME: 10 MINUTES / COOK TIME: 20 MINUTES/ SERVES 6

Ingredients

4 sweet potatoes, peeled and cubed
¼ cup almond milk
¼ cup extra-virgin olive oil
½ teaspoon sea salt
⅛ teaspoon freshly ground black pepper

Directions

Preparing the Ingredients

1.   In a large pot over high heat, combine the sweet potatoes with enough water to cover by 2 inches. Bring the water to a boil. Reduce the heat to medium and cover the pot. Cook for 15 to 20 minutes until the potatoes are soft.

2.   Drain the potatoes and return them to the dry pot off the heat. Add the almond milk, olive oil, sea salt, and pepper. With a potato masher, mash until smooth.
3.   Here are some alternative flavor combos to try with your sweet potatoes: Roasted Garlic: Mash in 6 roasted garlic cloves and 2 tablespoons chopped fresh chives. Orange: Replace the almond milk with ¼ cup unsweetened nonfat plain Greek yogurt, and add the zest and juice of 1 orange and ½ teaspoon ground nutmeg. Pineapple: Drain ½ cup canned crushed pineapple and warm it on the stove top or in the microwave. Stir the warmed pineapple into the hot rinsed potatoes.

No-Stir Polenta with Arugula, Figs, and Blue Cheese (Instant Pot)

PREP TIME: 10 MINUTES / COOK TIME: 40 MINUTES/ SERVES 4

Ingredients

1 cup coarse-ground cornmeal
½ cup oil-packed sun-dried tomatoes, chopped
1 teaspoon minced fresh thyme or ¼ teaspoon dried
½ teaspoon table salt
¼ teaspoon pepper
3 tablespoons extra-virgin olive oil, divided
2 ounces (2 cups) baby arugula
4 figs, cut into ½-inch-thick wedges
1 tablespoon balsamic vinegar
2 ounces blue cheese, crumbled (½ cup)
2 tablespoons pine nuts, toasted

Directions

1.   Arrange trivet included with Instant Pot in base of insert and add 1 cup water. Fold sheet of aluminum foil into 16 by 6-inch sling, then rest 1½-quart round soufflé dish in center of sling. Whisk 4 cups water, cornmeal, tomatoes, thyme, salt, and pepper together in bowl, then transfer mixture to soufflé dish. Using sling, lower soufflé dish into pot and onto trivet; allow narrow edges of sling to rest along sides of insert.
2.   Lock lid in place and close pressure release valve. Select high pressure cook function and cook for 40 minutes. Turn off Instant Pot and quick-release pressure. Carefully remove lid, allowing steam to escape away from you.
3.   Using sling, transfer soufflé dish to wire rack. Whisk 1 tablespoon oil into polenta, smoothing out any lumps. Let sit until thickened slightly, about 10 minutes. Season with salt and pepper to taste.
4.   Toss arugula and figs with vinegar and remaining 2 tablespoons oil in bowl, and season with salt and pepper to taste. Divide polenta among individual serving plates and top with arugula mixture, blue cheese, and pine nuts. Serve.

Brown Rice Pilaf with Golden Raisins

PREP TIME: 5 MINUTES / COOK TIME: 15 MINUTES/ SERVES 6

Ingredients

1 tablespoon extra-virgin olive oil
1 cup chopped onion (about ½ medium onion)
½ cup shredded carrot (about 1 medium carrot)
1 teaspoon ground cumin
½ teaspoon ground cinnamon
2 cups instant brown rice
1¾ cups 100% orange juice
¼ cup water
1 cup golden raisins
½ cup shelled pistachios
Chopped fresh chives (optional)
Directions
Preparing the Ingredients
1.   In a medium saucepan over medium-high heat, heat the oil. Add the onion and cook for 5 minutes, stirring frequently. Add the carrot, cumin, and cinnamon, and cook for 1 minute, stirring frequently. Stir in the rice, orange juice, and water. Bring to a boil, cover, then lower the heat to medium-low. Simmer for 7 minutes, or until the rice is cooked through and the liquid is absorbed. Stir in the raisins, pistachios, and chives (if using) and serve.

Tabbouleh

PREP TIME: 5 MINUTES / COOK TIME: 5 MINUTES / SERVES 6
Ingredients
2 cups cooked whole-wheat couscous, cooled completely
12 cherry tomatoes, quartered
6 scallions, white and green parts, minced
1 cucumber, peeled and chopped
½ cup fresh Italian parsley leaves, chopped
½ cup fresh mint leaves, chopped
Juice of 2 lemons
¼ cup extra-virgin olive oil
½ teaspoon sea salt
¼ teaspoon freshly ground black pepper
Directions
1.   **Preparing the Ingredients**
In a large bowl, combine the couscous, tomatoes, scallions, cucumber, parsley, and mint. Set aside.
In a small bowl, whisk the lemon juice, olive oil, sea salt, and pepper. Toss with the couscous mixture. Let sit for 1 hour before serving.
2.   **Cooking.** To make 2 cups cooked couscous: In a saucepan over high heat, bring 2 cups water or unsalted vegetable broth to a boil. Add 1 cup couscous, stir, turn off the heat, and cover the pot. After 5 minutes, uncover and fluff with a fork.

Brown Rice with Tomatoes and Chickpeas

PREP TIME: 5 MINUTES / COOK TIME: 35 MINUTES/ SERVES 6
Ingredients
12 ounces grape tomatoes, quartered
5 scallions, sliced thin
¼ cup minced fresh cilantro
4 teaspoons extra-virgin olive oil
1 tablespoon lime juice
Salt and pepper
2 red bell peppers, stemmed, seeded, and chopped fine
1 onion, chopped fine
1 cup long-grain brown rice, rinsed
4 garlic cloves, minced
Pinch saffron threads, crumbled
Pinch cayenne pepper
3¼ cups chicken or vegetable broth
2 (15-ounce) cans chickpeas, rinsed
Directions
1.   **Preparing the Ingredients**.
Combine tomatoes, scallions, cilantro, 2 teaspoons oil, and lime juice in bowl. Season with salt and pepper to taste; set aside for serving.
2.   **Cooking**
Heat remaining 2 teaspoons oil in large saucepan over medium-high heat until shimmering. Add bell peppers and onion and cook until softened and lightly browned, 8 to 10 minutes. Stir in rice, garlic, saffron, and cayenne and cook until fragrant, about 30 seconds.
Stir in broth and bring to simmer. Reduce heat to medium-low, cover, and simmer, stirring occasionally, for 25 minutes.
Stir in chickpeas, cover, and simmer until rice is tender and broth is almost completely absorbed, 25 to 30 minutes. Season with salt and pepper to taste. Serve, topping individual portions with tomato mixture.

Wild Mushroom Farrotto (Instant Pot)

PREP TIME: 30 MINUTES / COOK TIME: 12 MINUTES/ SERVES 4 TO 6
Ingredients
1½ cups whole farro
3 tablespoons extra-virgin olive oil, divided, plus extra for drizzling
12 ounces cremini or white mushrooms, trimmed and sliced thin
½ onion, chopped fine
½ teaspoon table salt
¼ teaspoon pepper
1 garlic clove, minced
¼ ounce dried porcini mushrooms, rinsed and chopped fine
2 teaspoons minced fresh thyme or ½ teaspoon dried
¼ cup dry white wine
2½ cups chicken or vegetable broth, plus extra as needed
2 ounces Parmesan cheese, grated (1 cup), plus extra for serving
2 teaspoons lemon juice
½ cup chopped fresh parsley
Directions
1.   Pulse farro in blender until about half of grains are broken into smaller pieces, about 6 pulses.
2.   Using highest sauté function, heat 2 tablespoons oil in Instant Pot until shimmering. Add cremini mushrooms, onion, salt, and pepper, partially

cover, and cook until mushrooms are softened and have released their liquid, about 5 minutes. Stir in farro, garlic, porcini mushrooms, and thyme and cook until fragrant, about 1 minute. Stir in wine and cook until nearly evaporated, about 30 seconds. Stir in broth.

3.　　　Lock lid in place and close pressure release valve. Select high pressure cook function and cook for 12 minutes. Turn off Instant Pot and quick-release pressure. Carefully remove lid, allowing steam to escape away from you. If necessary adjust consistency with extra hot broth, or continue to cook farrotto, using highest sauté function, stirring frequently, until proper consistency is achieved. (Farrotto should be slightly thickened, and spoon dragged along bottom of multicooker should leave trail that quickly fills in.) Add Parmesan and remaining 1 tablespoon oil and stir vigorously until farrotto becomes creamy. Stir in lemon juice and season with salt and pepper to taste. Sprinkle individual portions with parsley and extra Parmesan, and drizzle with extra oil before serving.

Lebanese Rice and Broken Noodles with Cabbage

PREP TIME: 5 MINUTES / COOK TIME: 25 MINUTES/ SERVES 6
Ingredients
1 tablespoon extra-virgin olive oil
1 cup (about 3 ounces) uncooked vermicelli or thin spaghetti, broken into 1- to 1½-inch pieces
3 cups shredded cabbage (about half a 14-ounce package of coleslaw mix or half a small head of cabbage)
3 cups low-sodium or no-salt-added vegetable broth
½ cup water
1 cup instant brown rice
2 garlic cloves
¼ teaspoon kosher or sea salt
⅛ to ¼ teaspoon crushed red pepper
½ cup loosely packed, coarsely chopped cilantro
Fresh lemon slices, for serving (optional)
Directions
Preparing the Ingredients
1.　　　In a large saucepan over medium-high heat, heat the oil. Add the pasta and cook for 3 minutes to toast, stirring often. Add the cabbage and cook for 4 minutes, stirring often. Add the broth, water, rice, garlic, salt, and crushed red pepper, and bring to a boil over high heat. Stir, cover, and reduce the heat to medium-low. Simmer for 10 minutes.
2.　　　Remove the pan from the heat, but do not lift the lid. Let sit for 5 minutes. Fish out the garlic cloves, mash them with a fork, then stir the garlic back into the rice. Stir in the cilantro. Serve with the lemon slices (if using).
3.　　　Ever wondered what to do with a leftover half head of cabbage or half a package of coleslaw mix? We love to cook it in a tablespoon of olive oil with chopped onion, then add it to canned soup,

scrambled eggs, tacos, or even leftover rice for stir-fried rice.

Orzo with Spinach and Feta

PREP TIME: 25 MINUTES / COOK TIME: NONE/ SERVES 6
Ingredients
6 cups fresh baby spinach, chopped
¼ cup scallions, white and green parts, chopped
1 (16-ounce) package orzo pasta, cooked according to package directions, rinsed, drained, and cooled
¾ cup crumbled feta cheese
¼ cup halved Kalamata olives
½ cup red wine vinegar
¼ cup extra-virgin olive oil
1½ teaspoons freshly squeezed lemon juice
Sea salt
Freshly ground black pepper
Directions
Preparing the Ingredients
1.　　　In a large bowl, combine the spinach, scallions, and cooled orzo.
2.　　　Sprinkle with the feta and olives.
3.　　　In a small bowl, whisk the vinegar, olive oil, and lemon juice. Season with sea salt and pepper.
4.　　　Add the dressing to the salad and gently toss to combine. Refrigerate until serving.

Rice Salad with Oranges, Olives, and Almonds

PREP TIME: 5 MINUTES / COOK TIME: NONE/ SERVES 4 TO 6
Ingredients
1½ cups basmati rice
Salt and pepper
2 oranges, plus ¼ teaspoon grated orange zest plus 1 tablespoon juice
2 tablespoons extra-virgin olive oil
2 teaspoons sherry vinegar
1 small garlic clove, minced
⅓ cup large pitted brine-cured green olives, chopped
⅓ cup slivered almonds, toasted
2 tablespoons minced fresh oregano
Directions
Preparing the Ingredients
1.　　　Bring 4 quarts water to boil in Dutch oven. Meanwhile, toast rice in 12-inch skillet over medium heat until faintly fragrant and some grains turn opaque, 5 to 8 minutes. Add rice and 1½ teaspoons salt to boiling water and cook, stirring occasionally, until rice is tender but not soft, about 15 minutes. Drain rice, spread onto rimmed baking sheet, and let cool completely, about 15 minutes.
2.　　　Cut away peel and pith from oranges. Holding fruit over bowl, use paring knife to slice between membranes to release segments. Whisk oil, vinegar, garlic, orange zest and juice, 1 teaspoon salt, and ½ teaspoon pepper together in large bowl. Add rice, orange segments, olives, almonds, and oregano, gently toss to combine, and let sit for 20 minutes.

Barley Salad with Lemon-Tahini Dressing (Instant Pot)

PREP TIME: 30 MINUTES / COOK TIME: 8 MINUTES/ MAKES 1½ CUP / SERVES 4 TO 6

Ingredients

1½ cups pearl barley
5 tablespoons extra-virgin olive oil, divided
1½ teaspoons table salt, for cooking barley
¼ cup tahini
1 teaspoon grated lemon zest plus ¼ cup juice (2 lemons)
1 tablespoon sumac, divided
1 garlic clove, minced
¾ teaspoon table salt
1 English cucumber, cut into ½-inch pieces
1 carrot, peeled and shredded
1 red bell pepper, stemmed, seeded, and chopped
4 scallions, sliced thin
2 tablespoons finely chopped jarred hot cherry peppers
¼ cup coarsely chopped fresh mint

Directions

1.   Combine 6 cups water, barley, 1 tablespoon oil, and 1½ teaspoons salt in Instant Pot. Lock lid in place and close pressure release valve. Select high pressure cook function and cook for 8 minutes. Turn off Instant Pot and let pressure release naturally for 15 minutes. Quick-release any remaining pressure, then carefully remove lid, allowing steam to escape away from you. Drain barley, spread onto rimmed baking sheet, and let cool completely, about 15 minutes.

2.   Meanwhile, whisk remaining ¼ cup oil, tahini, 2 tablespoons water, lemon zest and juice, 1 teaspoon sumac, garlic, and ¾ teaspoon salt in large bowl until combined; let sit for 15 minutes. Measure out and reserve ½ cup dressing for serving. Add barley, cucumber, carrot, bell pepper, scallions, and cherry peppers to bowl with dressing and gently toss to combine. Season with salt and pepper to taste. Transfer salad to serving dish and sprinkle with mint and remaining 2 teaspoons sumac. Serve, passing reserved dressing separately.

Lemon Farro Bowl with Avocado

PREP TIME: 5 MINUTES / COOK TIME: 25 MINUTES/ MAKES 1 CUP / SERVES 6

Ingredients

1 tablespoon plus 2 teaspoons extra-virgin olive oil, divided
1 cup chopped onion (about ½ medium onion)
2 garlic cloves, minced (about 1 teaspoon)
1 carrot, shredded (about 1 cup)
2 cups low-sodium or no-salt-added vegetable broth
1 cup (6 ounces) uncooked pearled or 10-minute farro
2 avocados, peeled, pitted, and sliced
1 small lemon
¼ teaspoon kosher or sea salt

Directions

Preparing the Ingredients

In a medium saucepan over medium-high heat, heat 1 tablespoon of oil. Add the onion and cook for 5 minutes, stirring occasionally. Add the garlic and carrot and cook for 1 minute, stirring frequently. Add the broth and farro, and bring to a boil over high heat. Lower the heat to medium-low, cover, and simmer for about 20 minutes or until the farro is plump and slightly chewy (al dente). Pour the farro into a serving bowl, and add the avocado slices.

Using a Microplane or citrus zester, zest the peel of the lemon directly into the bowl of farro.

Halve the lemon, and squeeze the juice out of both halves using a citrus juicer or your hands. Drizzle the remaining 2 teaspoons of oil over the bowl, and sprinkle with salt. Gently mix all the ingredients and serve. Have you noticed we add lemon juice or vinegar to many of our recipes? If you've ever made a dish, tasted it, and thought something was missing, that something might be acid. Acidic ingredients like citrus juices and vinegars bring sparkle to dishes and give them an additional layer of flavor beyond just adding more salt.

Cannellini Bean Salad (Instant Pot)

PREP TIME: 30 MINUTES / COOK TIME: 3 MINUTES, PLUS BRINING TIME/ SERVES 6 TO 8

Ingredients

1½ tablespoons table salt, for brining
1 pound (2½ cups) dried cannellini beans, picked over and rinsed
¼ cup extra-virgin olive oil, divided
¾ teaspoon table salt, divided
¼ cup tahini
3 tablespoons lemon juice
1 tablespoon ground dried Aleppo pepper, plus extra for sprinkling
8 ounces cherry tomatoes, halved
¼ red onion, sliced thin
½ cup fresh parsley leaves
1 recipe hard-cooked eggs, quartered (optional)
1 tablespoon toasted sesame seeds

Directions

Preparing the Ingredients

Dissolve 1½ tablespoons salt in 2 quarts cold water in large container. Add beans and soak at room temperature for at least 8 hours or up to 24 hours. Drain and rinse well. Add beans, 8 cups water, 1 tablespoon oil, and ½ teaspoon salt to Instant Pot. Lock lid in place and close pressure release valve. Select low pressure cook function and cook for 3 minutes. Turn off Instant Pot and quick-release pressure. Carefully remove lid, allowing steam to escape away from you.

Drain beans, rinse with cold water, and drain again. Meanwhile, whisk remaining 3 tablespoons oil, tahini, lemon juice, Aleppo pepper, 1 tablespoon water, and remaining ¼ teaspoon salt in large bowl until combined; let sit for 15 minutes.

Add beans, tomatoes, onion, and parsley and gently toss to combine. Season with salt and pepper to taste. Transfer salad to serving dish and arrange eggs on top, if using. Sprinkle with sesame seeds and extra Aleppo pepper to taste.

Barley Risotto with Parmesan

PREP TIME: 5 MINUTES / COOK TIME: 25 MINUTES/ SERVES 6

Ingredients

4 cups low-sodium or no-salt-added vegetable broth
1 tablespoon extra-virgin olive oil
1 cup chopped yellow onion (about ½ medium onion)
2 cups uncooked pearl barley
½ cup dry white wine
1 cup freshly grated Parmesan cheese (about 4 ounces), divided
¼ teaspoon kosher or sea salt
¼ teaspoon freshly ground black pepper
Fresh chopped chives and lemon wedges, for serving (optional)

Directions

Preparing the Ingredients

1.   Pour the broth into a medium saucepan and bring to a simmer.
2.   In a large stockpot over medium-high heat, heat the oil. Add the onion and cook for 8 minutes, stirring occasionally. Add the barley and cook for 2 minutes, stirring until the barley is toasted.
Pour in the wine and cook for about 1 minute, or until most of the liquid evaporates. Add 1 cup of warm broth to the pot and cook, stirring, for about 2 minutes, or until most of the liquid is absorbed. Add the remaining broth 1 cup at a time, cooking until each cup is absorbed (about 2 minutes each time) before adding the next. The last addition of broth will take a bit longer to absorb, about 4 minutes.
3.   Remove the pot from the heat, and stir in ½ cup of cheese, and the salt and pepper. Serve with the remaining cheese on the side, along with the chives and lemon wedges (if using).
4.   Pearled (quick) barley is not a whole grain, but it is high in protein and fiber and cooks in only 10 minutes, while whole-grain barley takes over an hour to cook. You may also find a new variety: whole hull-less barley, which takes about 40 minutes to cook.

French Lentils with Swiss Chard (Instant pot)

PREP TIME: 30 MINUTES / COOK TIME: 11 MINUTES/ MAKES 1 CUP / SERVES 6

Ingredients

2 tablespoons extra-virgin olive oil, plus extra for drizzling
12 ounces Swiss chard, stems chopped fine, leaves sliced into ½-inch-wide strips
1 onion, chopped fine
½ teaspoon table salt
2 garlic cloves, minced
1 teaspoon minced fresh thyme or ¼ teaspoon dried
2½ cups water
1 cup French green lentils, picked over and rinsed
3 tablespoons whole-grain mustard
½ teaspoon grated lemon zest plus 1 teaspoon juice

3 tablespoons sliced almonds, toasted
2 tablespoons chopped fresh parsley

Directions

1.   Using highest sauté function, heat oil in Instant Pot until shimmering. Add chard stems, onion, and salt and cook until vegetables are softened, about 5 minutes. Stir in garlic and thyme and cook until fragrant, about 30 seconds. Stir in water and lentils.
2.   Lock lid in place and close pressure release valve. Select high pressure cook function and cook for 11 minutes. Turn off Instant Pot and let pressure release naturally for 15 minutes. Quick-release any remaining pressure, then carefully remove lid, allowing steam to escape away from you.
3.   Stir chard leaves into lentils, 1 handful at a time, and let cook in residual heat until wilted, about 5 minutes. Stir in mustard and lemon zest and juice. Season with salt and pepper to taste. Transfer to serving dish, drizzle with extra oil, and sprinkle with almonds and parsley. Serve.

Garlic-Asparagus Israeli Couscous

PREP TIME: 5 MINUTES / COOK TIME: 25 MINUTES/ MAKES 1 CUP / SERVES 6

Ingredients

1 cup garlic-and-herb goat cheese (about 4 ounces)
1½ pounds asparagus spears, ends trimmed and stalks chopped into 1-inch pieces (about 2¾ to 3 cups chopped)
1 tablespoon extra-virgin olive oil
1 garlic clove, minced (about ½ teaspoon)
¼ teaspoon freshly ground black pepper
1¾ cups water
1 (8-ounce) box uncooked whole-wheat or regular Israeli couscous (about 1⅓ cups)
¼ teaspoon kosher or sea salt

Directions

1.   **Preparing the Ingredients**. Preheat the oven to 425°F. Put the goat cheese on the counter to bring to room temperature.
2.   In a large bowl, mix together the asparagus, oil, garlic, and pepper. Spread the asparagus on a large, rimmed baking sheet and roast for 10 minutes, stirring a few times.
Remove the pan from the oven, and spoon the asparagus into a large serving bowl. While the asparagus is roasting, in a medium saucepan, bring the water to a boil. Add the couscous and salt. Reduce the heat to medium-low, cover, and cook for 12 minutes, or until the water is absorbed.
3.   Pour the hot couscous into the bowl with the asparagus. Add the goat cheese, mix thoroughly until completely melted, and serve.
4.   Goat cheese melts into an instant creamy sauce when mixed with hot grains, as in this recipe. Ricotta cheese is an alternative here, along with adding in some fresh chopped herbs such as rosemary, basil, and/or oregano.

to pasta and toss to combine. Season with salt and pepper to taste and adjust consistency with reserved cooking water as needed.

Penne and Fresh Tomato Sauce with Spinach and Feta

PREP TIME: 10 MINUTES / COOK TIME: 15 MINUTES/ SERVES 6

Ingredients
3 tablespoons extra-virgin olive oil
2 garlic cloves, minced
3 pounds ripe tomatoes, cored, peeled, seeded, and cut into ½-inch pieces
5 ounces (5 cups) baby spinach
1 pound penne
Salt and pepper
2 tablespoons chopped fresh mint or oregano
2 tablespoons lemon juice
Sugar
4 ounces feta cheese, crumbled (1 cup)

Directions
Preparing the Ingredients
1.   Cook 2 tablespoons oil and garlic in 12-inch skillet over medium heat, stirring often, until garlic turns golden but not brown, about 3 minutes. Stir in tomatoes and cook until tomato pieces begin to lose their shape, about 8 minutes. Stir in spinach, 1 handful at a time, and cook until spinach is wilted and tomatoes have made chunky sauce, about 2 minutes.
2.   Meanwhile, bring 4 quarts water to boil in large pot. Add pasta and 1 tablespoon salt and cook, stirring often, until al dente. Reserve ½ cup cooking water, then drain pasta and return it to pot.
3.   Stir mint, lemon juice, ¼ teaspoon salt, and ⅛ teaspoon pepper into sauce and season with sugar to taste.
4.   Add sauce and remaining 1 tablespoon oil to pasta and toss to combine. Season with salt and pepper to taste and adjust consistency with reserved cooking water as needed. Serve, passing feta separately.

Couscous with Chicken, Fennel, and Peppers (Instant Pot)

PREP TIME: 30 MINUTES / COOK TIME: 4 MINUTES/ SERVES 4 TO 6

Ingredients
2 teaspoons ground fenugreek
½ teaspoon table salt
½ teaspoon pepper
½ teaspoon ground cardamom
¼ cup extra-virgin olive oil, divided, plus extra for serving
1 pound ground chicken
1 onion, chopped
1 fennel bulb, 2 tablespoons fronds chopped, stalks discarded, bulb halved, cored, and cut into ½-inch pieces
1½ cups pearl couscous

3 garlic cloves, minced
2¼ cups chicken broth
1 cup jarred roasted red peppers, sliced ¼ inch thick
¼ cup walnuts, toasted and chopped coarse
2 tablespoons chopped fresh parsley

Directions
Preparing the Ingredients
1.   Combine fenugreek, salt, pepper, and cardamom in bowl. Using highest sauté function, heat 2 tablespoons oil in Instant Pot until shimmering. Add chicken and 1 teaspoon spice mixture and cook, breaking up any large chicken pieces with wooden spoon, until no longer pink, 5 to 7 minutes. Using slotted spoon, transfer chicken to separate bowl.
2.   Add onion, fennel pieces, and remaining 2 tablespoons oil to fat left in pot and cook, using highest sauté function, until vegetables are softened, 6 to 8 minutes. Add couscous and cook, stirring frequently, until lightly browned, about 3 minutes. Stir in garlic and remaining spice mixture and cook until fragrant, about 1 minute.
3.   Stir in broth, scraping up any browned bits. Lock lid in place and close pressure release valve. Select high pressure cook function and cook for 4 minutes. Turn off Instant Pot and quick-release pressure. Carefully remove lid, allowing steam to escape away from you.
4.   Stir in red peppers and chicken and any accumulated juices. Season with salt and pepper to taste. Transfer to serving dish. Sprinkle with walnuts, parsley, and fennel fronds, and drizzle with extra oil.

White Clam Pizza Pie

PREP TIME: 10 MINUTES / COOK TIME: 20 MINUTES/ SERVES 4

Ingredients
1 pound refrigerated fresh pizza dough
Nonstick cooking spray
2 tablespoons extra-virgin olive oil, divided
2 garlic cloves, minced (about 1 teaspoon)
½ teaspoon crushed red pepper
1 (10-ounce) can whole baby clams, drained, ⅓ cup of juice reserved
¼ cup dry white wine
All-purpose flour, for dusting
1 cup diced fresh or shredded mozzarella cheese (about 4 ounces)
1 tablespoon grated Pecorino Romano or Parmesan cheese
1 tablespoon chopped fresh flat-leaf (Italian) parsley

Directions
Preparing the Ingredients
1.   Preheat the oven to 500°F. Take the pizza dough out of the refrigerator. Coat a large, rimmed baking sheet with nonstick cooking spray.
2.   In a large skillet over medium heat, heat 1½ tablespoons of the oil. Add the garlic and crushed red pepper and cook for 1 minute, stirring frequently to prevent the garlic from burning. Add the reserved clam juice and wine. Bring to a boil over high heat.

Reduce to medium heat so the sauce is just simmering and cook for 10 minutes, stirring occasionally. The sauce will cook down and thicken.

3.	Stir in the clams and cook for 3 minutes, stirring occasionally.

While the sauce is cooking, on a lightly floured surface, form the pizza dough into a 12-inch circle or into a 10-by-12-inch rectangle with a rolling pin or by stretching with your hands. Place the dough on the prepared baking sheet. Brush the dough with the remaining ½ tablespoon of oil. Set aside until the clam sauce is ready.

4.	Spread the clam sauce over the prepared dough within ½ inch of the edge. Top with the mozzarella cheese, then sprinkle with the Pecorino Romano.

Bake for 10 minutes, or until the crust starts to brown around the edges. Remove the pizza from the oven and slide onto a wooden cutting board. Top with the parsley, cut into eight pieces with a pizza cutter or a sharp knife, and serve.

Sun-Dried Tomato and Artichoke Pizza

PREP TIME: 25 MINUTES / COOK TIME: 25 MINUTES/ SERVES 6

Ingredients

¾ cup whole-wheat flour, plus more for flouring the work surface
¾ cup all-purpose flour
1 package quick-rising yeast
¾ teaspoon sea salt
⅔ cup hot water (120°F to 125°F)
2 tablespoons extra-virgin olive oil
¼ teaspoon honey
Nonstick cooking spray
2 tablespoons extra-virgin olive oil
½ onion, minced
3 garlic cloves, minced
1 (14-ounce) can crushed tomatoes
1 tablespoon dried oregano
1 cup oil-packed sun-dried tomatoes, rinsed
2 cups frozen artichoke hearts
¼ cup (about 2 ounces) grated Asiago cheese

Directions

Preparing the Ingredients

1.	In a medium bowl, whisk the whole-wheat and all-purpose flours, yeast, and salt. In a small bowl, whisk the hot water, olive oil, and honey. Mix the liquids into the flour mixture and stir until sticky ball forms. Turn the dough out onto a floured surface and knead for 5 minutes. Coat a sheet of plastic wrap with cooking spray and cover the dough. Let rest for 10 minutes. Roll the dough into a 13-inch circle.

2.	In a saucepan over medium-high heat, heat the olive oil until it shimmers. Add the onion and cook for 5 minutes, stirring occasionally. Add the garlic and cook for 30 seconds, stirring constantly. Stir in the tomatoes and oregano. Bring to a simmer. Reduce the heat to medium-low and simmer for 5 minutes more.

3.	Preheat the oven to 500°F (or the hottest setting). If you have a pizza stone, place it in the oven as it preheats.

In a thin layer, spread the sauce over the rolled dough. Top the sauce with the artichoke hearts and sun-dried tomatoes. Sprinkle the cheese lightly over the top. Place the pizza on the stone (or directly on the rack) and bake for 10 to 15 minutes until the crust is golden. If you have a food processor or stand mixer, use it to make the crust and save yourself a lot of time and elbow grease. Add the dry ingredients, mix with the food processor or mixer, and with the mixer running, slowly add the wet ingredients until a sticky ball forms. In a food processor, process on high speed for 1 minute to knead. In a stand mixer, use the dough hook on high speed for 5 minutes to knead.

Roasted Broccolini with Garlic and Romano

PREP TIME: 5 MINUTES / COOK TIME: 10 MINUTES/ SERVES 2

Ingredients

1 bunch broccolini (about 5 ounces)
1 tablespoon olive oil
½ teaspoon garlic powder
¼ teaspoon salt
2 tablespoons grated Romano cheese

Directions

1.	**Preparing the Ingredients**. Preheat the oven to 400°F and set the oven rack to the middle position. Line a sheet pan with parchment paper or foil. Slice the tough ends off the broccolini and place in a medium bowl. Add the olive oil, garlic powder, and salt and toss to combine. Arrange broccolini on the lined sheet pan.

2.	**Cooking.** Roast for 7 minutes, flipping pieces over halfway through the roasting time. Remove the pan from the oven and sprinkle the cheese over the broccolini. With a pair of tongs, carefully flip the pieces over to coat all sides. Return to the oven for another 2 to 3 minutes, or until the cheese melts and starts to turn golden.

Toasted Orzo with Shrimp and Feta

PREP TIME: 30 MINUTES / COOK TIME: 30 MINUTES/ SERVES 4 TO 6

Ingredients

1 pound large shrimp (26 to 30 per pound), peeled and deveined
1 tablespoon grated lemon zest plus 1 tablespoon juice
¼ teaspoon table salt
¼ teaspoon pepper
2 tablespoons extra-virgin olive oil, plus extra for serving
1 onion, chopped fine
2 garlic cloves, minced
2 cups orzo
2 cups chicken broth, plus extra as needed
1¼ cups water

½ cup pitted kalamata olives, chopped coarse
1 ounce feta cheese, crumbled (¼ cup), plus extra for serving
1 tablespoon chopped fresh dill
Directions
1.   Toss shrimp with lemon zest, salt, and pepper in bowl; refrigerate until ready to use. Using highest sauté function, heat oil in Instant Pot until shimmering. Add onion and cook until softened, about 5 minutes. Stir in garlic and cook until fragrant, about 30 seconds. Add orzo and cook, stirring frequently, until orzo is coated with oil and lightly browned, about 5 minutes. Stir in broth and water, scraping up any browned bits.
2.   Lock lid in place and close pressure release valve. Select high pressure cook function and cook for 2 minutes. Turn off Instant Pot and quick-release pressure. Carefully remove lid, allowing steam to escape away from you. Stir shrimp, olives, and feta into orzo. Cover and let sit until shrimp are opaque throughout, 5 to 7 minutes. Adjust consistency with extra hot broth as needed. Stir in dill and lemon juice, and season with salt and pepper to taste. Sprinkle individual portions with extra feta and drizzle with extra oil before serving.

Mediterranean Veggie Pizza with Pourable Thin Crust

PREP TIME: 15 MINUTES / COOK TIME: 15 MINUTES / SERVES 4
Ingredients
Nonstick cooking spray
3 tablespoons cornmeal
1 cup white whole-wheat flour or regular whole-wheat flour
½ cup all-purpose flour
1 tablespoon dried oregano, crushed between your fingers
¼ teaspoon kosher or sea salt
1 cup plus 2 tablespoons 2% milk
2 large eggs, beaten
1 large bell pepper, sliced into ⅛-inch-thick rounds
1 (2.25-ounce) can sliced olives, any type of green or black, drained (about ½ cup)
3 whole canned artichoke hearts, drained and quartered
⅓ cup thinly sliced red onion (about ⅙ onion)
½ cup feta cheese (about 2 ounces), crumbled
Extra-virgin olive oil, for topping (optional)
Directions
Preparing the Ingredients
1.   Place one oven rack about 4 inches below the broiler element. Preheat the oven to 400°F. Spray a large, rimmed baking sheet with nonstick cooking spray. Sprinkle it with the cornmeal and set aside.
2.   In a large bowl, whisk together the flours, oregano, and salt. In a small bowl, whisk together the milk and eggs; mix into the flour mixture until well combined.

3.   Pour the mixture onto the prepared baking sheet. Using a rubber scraper, carefully spread the batter evenly to the corners of the pan. Arrange the bell pepper slices evenly over the batter.
4.   Bake on any oven rack for 10 to 12 minutes, or until the crust is dry on top. Remove the pizza crust from the oven.
5.   Turn the oven broiler to high.
6.   Top the pizza crust with the olives, artichoke hearts, and onion. Top with the feta cheese. Place the pizza on the upper oven rack under the broiler. Broil until the cheese is melted and golden, rotating the pan halfway through and watching carefully to prevent burning. Top with a drizzle of olive oil.

Pizza with Arugula and Balsamic Glaze

PREP TIME: 30 MINUTES / COOK TIME: 20 MINUTES / SERVES 6
Ingredients
¾ cup whole-wheat flour, plus more for flouring the work surface
¾ cup all-purpose flour
1 package quick-rising yeast
¾ teaspoon sea salt
⅔ cup hot water (120° to 125°F)
2 tablespoons extra-virgin olive oil
¼ teaspoon honey
Nonstick cooking spray
½ cup balsamic vinegar
2 tablespoons honey
4 cups arugula
2 tablespoons extra-virgin olive oil
½ teaspoon sea salt
⅛ teaspoon freshly ground black pepper
Directions
Preparing the Ingredients
1.   In a medium bowl, whisk the whole-wheat and all-purpose flours, yeast, and sea salt.
In a small bowl, whisk the hot water, olive oil, and honey.
2.   Mix the liquids into the flour mixture and stir until a sticky ball forms.
3.   Turn the dough out onto a floured surface and knead for 5 minutes.
Coat a sheet of plastic wrap with cooking spray and cover the dough. Let rest for 10 minutes.
4.   Roll the dough into a 13-inch circle.
5.   In a small saucepan over medium-high heat, stir together the vinegar and honey. Simmer for about 5 minutes, stirring occasionally, until syrupy.
6.   Preheat the oven to 500°F (or the hottest setting).
If you have a pizza stone, place it in the oven as it preheats.
Place the pizza crust on the stone (or directly on the rack) and bake for 10 to 15 minutes, until the crust is golden.
7.   In a medium bowl, toss the arugula with the olive oil, sea salt, and pepper. Spread the mixture

over the warm crust and drizzle with the balsamic glaze.

Make the dough ahead of time and refrigerate or freeze it, uncooked. Wrap the dough tightly in oiled plastic wrap to refrigerate (for up to 1 day) or freeze (for up to 3 months). Thaw frozen dough in the refrigerator overnight, and allow the cold dough to stand at room temperature for 30 minutes before using.

Roasted Brussels Sprouts with Delicata Squash and Balsamic Glaze

PREP TIME: 10 MINUTES / COOK TIME: 30 MINUTES / SERVES 2

Ingredients

½ pound Brussels sprouts, ends trimmed and outer leaves removed
1 medium delicata squash, halved lengthwise, seeded, and cut into 1-inch pieces
1 cup fresh cranberries
2 teaspoons olive oil
Salt
Freshly ground black pepper
½ cup balsamic vinegar
2 tablespoons roasted pumpkin seeds
2 tablespoons fresh pomegranate arils (seeds)

Directions

Preparing the Ingredients

1.   Preheat oven to 400°F and set the rack to the middle position. Line a sheet pan with parchment paper.

Combine the Brussels sprouts, squash, and cranberries in a large bowl. Drizzle with olive oil, and season liberally with salt and pepper. Toss well to coat and arrange in a single layer on the sheet pan. Roast for 30 minutes, turning vegetables halfway through, or until Brussels sprouts turn brown and crisp in spots and squash has golden-brown spots.

2.   While vegetables are roasting, prepare the balsamic glaze by simmering the vinegar for 10 to 12 minutes, or until mixture has reduced to about ¼ cup and turns a syrupy consistency.

Remove the vegetables from the oven, drizzle with balsamic syrup, and sprinkle with pumpkin seeds and pomegranate arils before serving.

3.   When fresh cranberries are in season, grab a few extra bags and store them in the freezer. They'll last for an entire year. Look for pomegranate arils in the prepared foods area of your grocery store produce section.

Triple-Green Pasta

PREP TIME: 5 MINUTES / COOK TIME: 15 MINUTES / SERVES 4

Ingredients

8 ounces uncooked penne
1 tablespoon extra-virgin olive oil
2 garlic cloves, minced (1 teaspoon)
¼ teaspoon crushed red pepper

2 cups chopped fresh flat-leaf (Italian) parsley, including stems
5 cups loosely packed baby spinach (about 5 ounces)
¼ teaspoon ground nutmeg
¼ teaspoon freshly ground black pepper
¼ teaspoon kosher or sea salt
⅓ cup Castelvetrano olives (or other green olives), pitted and sliced (about 12)
⅓ cup grated Pecorino Romano or Parmesan cheese (about 1 ounce)

Directions

Preparing the Ingredients

1.   In a large stockpot, cook the pasta according to the package directions, but boil 1 minute less than instructed. Drain the pasta, and save ¼ cup of the cooking water.

2.   While the pasta is cooking, in a large skillet over medium heat, heat the oil. Add the garlic and crushed red pepper, and cook for 30 seconds, stirring constantly. Add the parsley and cook for 1 minute, stirring constantly. Add the spinach, nutmeg, pepper, and salt, and cook for 3 minutes, stirring occasionally, until the spinach is wilted.

3.   Add the pasta and the reserved ¼ cup pasta water to the skillet. Stir in the olives, and cook for about 2 minutes, until most of the pasta water has been absorbed. Remove from the heat, stir in the cheese, and serve.

4.   Besides the multitude of pasta shapes on the market, there's also a huge variety when it comes to both wheat-based and wheat-free pastas. Whole-wheat, whole-grain, chickpea, lentil, quinoa, or a combination of grains and beans are all options. Our recommendation is to use the type of pasta you enjoy and pair it with vegetables, fish and seafood, and lean proteins, but also experiment with a new variety from time to time.

Pizza with Red Bell Peppers, Basil, Arugula, and Caramelized Onion

PREP TIME: 30 MINUTES / COOK TIME: 30 MINUTES / SERVES 6

Ingredients

¾ cup whole-wheat flour, plus more for flouring the work surface
¾ cup all-purpose flour
1 package quick-rising yeast
¾ teaspoon sea salt
⅔ cup hot water (120° to 125°F)
2 tablespoons extra-virgin olive oil
¼ teaspoon honey
Nonstick cooking spray
2 tablespoons extra-virgin olive oil
1 onion, thinly sliced
½ teaspoon sea salt
2 tablespoons extra-virgin olive oil
½ red bell pepper, sliced
½ cup grated mozzarella cheese
1 cup arugula
¼ cup chopped fresh basil leaves

¼ cup shaved Asiago cheese

Directions

1.   Preparing the Ingredients

In a medium bowl, whisk the whole-wheat and all-purpose flours, yeast, and salt. In a small bowl, whisk the hot water, olive oil, and honey. Mix the liquids into the flour mixture and stir until a sticky ball forms. Turn the dough out onto a floured surface and knead for 5 minutes. Coat a sheet of plastic wrap with cooking spray and cover the dough. Let rest for 10 minutes. Roll the dough into a 13-inch circle.

2.   Cooking

In a large skillet over medium heat, heat the olive oil. Add the onion and salt. Cook for 3 minutes, stirring occasionally. Reduce the heat to medium-low. Cook for 20 to 35 minutes, stirring occasionally, until the onion is browned and caramelized. Preheat the oven to 500°F (or the hottest setting). If you have a pizza stone, place it in the oven as it preheats. Brush the crust with olive oil. Spread the onion over the crust and top with the red bell pepper and mozzarella cheese. Place the pizza on the stone (or directly on the rack) and bake for 15 to 20 minutes until the crust is browned.

Remove from the oven. Top with the arugula, basil, and Asiago cheese.

Coriander-Cumin Roasted Carrots

PREP TIME: 10 MINUTES / COOK TIME: 20 MINUTES / SERVES 2

Ingredients

½ pound rainbow carrots (about 4)
2 tablespoons fresh orange juice
1 tablespoon honey
½ teaspoon coriander
Pinch salt

Directions

1.   Preparing the Ingredients

Preheat oven to 400°F and set the oven rack to the middle position. Peel the carrots and cut them lengthwise into slices of even thickness. Place them in a large bowl. In a small bowl, mix together the orange juice, honey, coriander, and salt. Pour the orange juice mixture over the carrots and toss well to coat. Spread carrots onto a baking dish in a single layer.

2.   Cooking

Roast for 15 to 20 minutes, or until fork-tender. If you can't find rainbow carrots, substitute regular orange carrots or parsnips.

No-Drain Pasta Alla Norma

PREP TIME: 5 MINUTES / COOK TIME: 25 MINUTES / SERVES 6

Ingredients

1 medium globe eggplant (about 1 pound), cut into ¾-inch cubes
1 tablespoon extra-virgin olive oil
1 cup chopped onion (about ½ medium onion)
8 ounces uncooked thin spaghetti

1 (15-ounce) container part-skim ricotta cheese
3 Roma tomatoes, chopped (about 2 cups)
2 garlic cloves, minced (about 1 teaspoon)
¼ teaspoon kosher or sea salt
½ cup loosely packed fresh basil leaves
Grated Parmesan cheese, for serving (optional)

Directions

Preparing the Ingredients

**1.   Lay three paper towels on a large plate, and pile the cubed eggplant on top. (Don't cover the eggplant.) Microwave the eggplant on high for 5 minutes to dry and partially cook it.

**2.   In a large stockpot over medium-high heat, heat the oil.

Add the eggplant and the onion and cook for 5 minutes, stirring occasionally. Add the spaghetti, ricotta, tomatoes, garlic, and salt. Cover with water by a ½ inch (about 4 cups of water).

Cook uncovered for 12 to 15 minutes, or until the pasta is just al dente (tender with a bite), stirring occasionally to prevent the pasta from sticking together or sticking to the bottom of the pot.

**3.   Remove the pot from the heat and let the pasta stand for 3 more minutes to absorb more liquid while you tear the basil into pieces. Sprinkle the basil over the pasta and gently stir. Serve with Parmesan cheese, if desired.

Flatbread with Olive Tapenade

PREP TIME: 30 MINUTES (PLUS 1 HOUR TO RISE) / COOK TIME: 5 MINUTES / SERVES 6

Ingredients

¾ cup warm water (120°F to 125°F)
1 tablespoon honey
1 package quick-rising yeast
¾ cup whole-wheat flour, plus more for dusting the work surface
¼ cup all-purpose flour
½ teaspoon sea salt
1 tablespoon extra-virgin olive oil
1 cup black olives, pitted and chopped
1 cup green olives, pitted and chopped
2 roasted red pepper slices, chopped
1 tablespoon capers, drained and rinsed
1 garlic clove, minced
1 tablespoon chopped fresh basil leaves
1 tablespoon chopped fresh oregano leaves
¼ cup extra-virgin olive oil

Directions

Preparing the Ingredients

**1.   In a small bowl, whisk the water, honey, and yeast. Let stand for about 5 minutes, covered with a clean kitchen towel, until the yeast foams. In a large bowl, whisk the whole-wheat and all-purpose flours and sea salt. Add the yeast mixture and stir until a ball forms. Turn the dough out onto a floured surface and knead for about 5 minutes until smooth.

**2.   Brush a bowl with olive oil. Add the dough and turn to coat with the oil.

Cover and place in a warm spot to rise for about 1 hour until doubled. Preheat the oven to 450°F. If you have a pizza stone, place it in the oven as it preheats. Split the dough into 6 portions. Roll each into a thin oblong shape, ¼ to ½ inch thick. Bake the flatbreads on the pizza stone (or directly on the rack) for about 5 minutes until browned. In a food processor or blender, combine the black and green olives, roasted pepper, capers, garlic, basil, oregano, and olive oil. Process for 10 to 20 (1-second) pulses until coarsely chopped.

3.   Make the tapenade ahead of time and store, tightly sealed, in the refrigerator for up to 1 week. The cooked flatbread will keep, tightly sealed, for up to 4 days.

Garlic and Herb Roasted Grape Tomatoes

PREP TIME: 10 MINUTES / COOK TIME: 45 MINUTES / SERVES 2

Ingredients
1 pint grape tomatoes
10 whole garlic cloves, skins removed
¼ cup olive oil
½ teaspoon salt
1 fresh rosemary sprig
1 fresh thyme sprig

Directions
Preparing the Ingredients
1.   Preheat oven to 350°F. Toss tomatoes, garlic cloves, oil, salt, and herb sprigs in a baking dish. Roast tomatoes until they are soft and begin to caramelize, about 45 minutes.
Remove herbs before serving.
2.   To peel many garlic cloves quickly, place them in a large bowl with a lid or a jar and shake them vigorously. The skins should fall off most of them.

Zucchini With Bow Ties

PREP TIME: 5 MINUTES / COOK TIME: 25 MINUTES / SERVES 4

Ingredients
3 tablespoons extra-virgin olive oil
2 garlic cloves, minced (about 1 teaspoon)
3 large or 4 medium zucchini, diced (about 4 cups)
½ teaspoon freshly ground black pepper
¼ teaspoon kosher or sea salt
½ cup 2% milk
¼ teaspoon ground nutmeg
8 ounces uncooked farfalle (bow ties) or other small pasta shape
½ cup grated Parmesan or Romano cheese (about 2 ounces)
1 tablespoon freshly squeezed lemon juice (from ½ medium lemon)

Directions
Preparing the Ingredients
1.   In a large skillet over medium heat, heat the oil. Add the garlic and cook for 1 minute, stirring frequently. Add the zucchini, pepper, and salt. Stir

well, cover, and cook for 15 minutes, stirring once or twice. In a small, microwave-safe bowl, warm the milk in the microwave on high for 30 seconds. Stir the milk and nutmeg into the skillet and cook uncovered for another 5 minutes, stirring occasionally.
While the zucchini is cooking, in a large stockpot, cook the pasta according to the package directions. Drain the pasta in a colander, saving about 2 tablespoons of pasta water.
Add the pasta and pasta water to the skillet. Mix everything together and remove from the heat. Stir in the cheese and lemon juice and serve.
2.   Save about ¼ to ½ cup of the starchy water before draining your cooked pasta. Add it to your sauce a few tablespoons at a time to thicken it up. Also, toss the pasta into the sauce right after draining to allow it to soak up more of the flavors of the sauce.

Roasted Cauliflower With Lemon Tahini Sauce

PREP TIME: 10 MINUTES / COOK TIME: 20 MINUTES / SERVES 2

Ingredients
½ large head cauliflower, stemmed and broken into florets (about 3 cups)
1 tablespoon olive oil
2 tablespoons tahini
2 tablespoons freshly squeezed lemon juice
1 teaspoon harissa paste
Pinch salt

Directions
Preparing the Ingredients
1.   Preheat the oven to 400°F and set the rack to the lowest position. Line a sheet pan with parchment paper or foil.
Toss the cauliflower florets with the olive oil in a large bowl and transfer to the sheet pan. Reserve the bowl to make the tahini sauce.
2.   Roast the cauliflower for 15 minutes, turning it once or twice, until it starts to turn golden. In the same bowl, combine the tahini, lemon juice, harissa, and salt.
3.   When the cauliflower is tender, remove it from the oven and toss it with the tahini sauce. Return to the sheet pan and roast for 5 minutes more.

Roasted Asparagus Caprese Pasta

PREP TIME: 5 MINUTES / COOK TIME: 25 MINUTES / SERVES 6

Ingredients
8 ounces uncooked small pasta, like orecchiette (little ears) or farfalle (bow ties)
1½ pounds fresh asparagus, ends trimmed and stalks chopped into 1-inch pieces (about 3 cups)
1 pint grape tomatoes, halved (about 1½ cups)
2 tablespoons extra-virgin olive oil
¼ teaspoon freshly ground black pepper
¼ teaspoon kosher or sea salt

2 cups fresh mozzarella, drained and cut into bite-size pieces (about 8 ounces)
⅓ cup torn fresh basil leaves
2 tablespoons balsamic vinegar

Directions

Preparing the Ingredients

1. Preheat the oven to 400°F.
2. In a large stockpot, cook the pasta according to the package directions. Drain, reserving about ¼ cup of the pasta water.
3. While the pasta is cooking, in a large bowl, toss the asparagus, tomatoes, oil, pepper, and salt together. Spread the mixture onto a large, rimmed baking sheet and bake for 15 minutes, stirring twice as it cooks.
4. Remove the vegetables from the oven, and add the cooked pasta to the baking sheet. Mix with a few tablespoons of pasta water to help the sauce become smoother and the saucy vegetables stick to the pasta.
5. Gently mix in the mozzarella and basil. Drizzle with the balsamic vinegar. Serve from the baking sheet or pour the pasta into a large bowl.

White Beans With Rosemary, Sage, And Garlic

PREP TIME: 10 MINUTES / COOK TIME: 10 MINUTES / SERVES 2

Ingredients
1 tablespoon olive oil
2 garlic cloves, minced
1 (15-ounce) can white cannellini beans, drained and rinsed
¼ teaspoon dried sage
1 teaspoon minced fresh rosemary (from 1 sprig) plus 1 whole fresh rosemary sprig
½ cup low-sodium chicken stock
Salt

Directions

Preparing the Ingredients

1. Heat the olive oil in a sauté pan over medium-high heat. Add the garlic and sauté for 30 seconds. Add the beans, sage, minced and whole rosemary, and chicken stock and bring the mixture to a boil.
2. Reduce the heat to medium and simmer the beans for 10 minutes, or until most of the liquid is evaporated. If desired, mash some of the beans with a fork to thicken them.
3. Season with salt. Remove the rosemary sprig before serving

Canned beans are one of the best convenience foods to keep on hand. When buying them, look for cans with no salt added so that you can control the amount of sodium in your dish.

DESSERTS AND SWEETS

Flourless Chocolate Brownies with Raspberry Balsamic Sauce

PREP TIME: 10 MINUTES, PLUS 5 MINUTES TO COOL / COOK TIME: 20 MINUTES/ SERVES 2

Ingredients

¼ cup good-quality balsamic vinegar
1 cup frozen raspberries
½ cup black beans with no added salt, rinsed
1 large egg
1 tablespoon olive oil
½ teaspoon vanilla extract
4 tablespoons unsweetened cocoa powder
¼ cup sugar
¼ teaspoon baking powder
Pinch salt
¼ cup dark chocolate chips

Directions

1.   Preparing the Ingredients

Combine the balsamic vinegar and raspberries in a saucepan and bring the mixture to a boil. Reduce the heat to medium and let the sauce simmer for 15 minutes, or until reduced to ½ cup. If desired, strain the seeds and set the sauce aside until the brownie is ready.

To make the brownie

Preheat the oven to 350°F and set the rack to the middle position. Grease two 8-ounce ramekins and place them on a baking sheet. In a food processor, combine the black beans, egg, olive oil, and vanilla. Purée the mixture for 1 to 2 minutes, or until it's smooth and the beans are completely broken down. Scrape down the sides of the bowl a few times to make sure everything is well-incorporated. Add the cocoa powder, sugar, baking powder, and salt and purée again to combine the dry ingredients, scraping down the sides of the bowl as needed. Stir the chocolate chips into the batter by hand. Reserve a few if you like, to sprinkle over the top of the brownies when they come out of the oven.

2.   Bake

Pour the brownies into the prepared ramekins and bake for 15 minutes, or until firm. The center will look slightly undercooked. If you prefer a firmer brownie, leave it in the oven for another 5 minutes, or until a toothpick inserted in the middle comes out clean.

Remove the brownies from the oven. If desired, sprinkle any remaining chocolate chips over the top and let them melt into the warm brownies. Let the brownies cool for a few minutes and top with warm raspberry sauce to serve.

This warm raspberry-balsamic sauce is delicious served over a scoop of vanilla, chocolate, or coconut gelato for a quick no-bake dessert.

Chilled Dark Chocolate Fruit Kebabs

PREP TIME: 10 MINUTES / CHILL TIME: 20 MINUTES/ SERVES 6

Ingredients

12 strawberries, hulled
12 cherries, pitted
24 seedless red or green grapes
24 blueberries
8 ounces dark chocolate

Directions

1.   Preparing the Ingredients

Line a large, rimmed baking sheet with parchment paper. On your work surface, lay out six 12-inch wooden skewers.

Thread the fruit onto the skewers, following this pattern: 1 strawberry, 1 cherry, 2 grapes, 2 blueberries, 1 strawberry, 1 cherry, 2 grapes, and 2 blueberries (or vary according to taste!). Place the kebabs on the prepared baking sheet.

**2.   **In a medium, microwave-safe bowl, heat the chocolate in the microwave for 1 minute on high. Stir until the chocolate is completely melted. Spoon the melted chocolate into a small plastic sandwich bag. Twist the bag closed right above the chocolate, and snip the corner of the bag off with scissors. Squeeze the bag to drizzle lines of chocolate over the kebabs.

**3.   **Place the sheet in the freezer and chill for 20 minutes before serving.

Honey Ricotta with Espresso and Chocolate Chips

PREP TIME: 5 MINUTES / COOK TIME: NONE/ SERVES 2

Ingredients

8 ounces ricotta cheese
2 tablespoons honey
2 tablespoons espresso, chilled or room temperature
1 teaspoon dark chocolate chips or chocolate shavings

Directions

Preparing the Ingredients

1.   In a medium bowl, whip together the ricotta cheese and honey until light and smooth, 4 to 5 minutes.

2.   Spoon the ricotta cheese–honey mixture evenly into 2 dessert bowls. Drizzle 1 tablespoon espresso into each dish and sprinkle with chocolate chips or shavings.

3.   Regular or decaf black coffee can be used in place of the espresso.

Lemon and Watermelon Granita

PREP TIME: 10 MINUTES (PLUS 3 HOURS TO FREEZE) / COOK TIME: NONE/ MAKES ½ CUP / SERVES 4

Ingredients

4 cups watermelon cubes
¼ cup honey
¼ cup freshly squeezed lemon juice

Directions
Preparing the Ingredients
1.　　In a blender, combine the watermelon, honey, and lemon juice. Purée all the ingredients, then pour into a 9-by-9-by-2-inch baking pan and place in the freezer.
Every 30 to 60 minutes, run a fork across the frozen surface to fluff and create ice flakes. Freeze for about 3 hours total and serve.
2.　　Leftovers tip: Serve leftovers like Italian ice, scraping it into cups with a spoon, or give it a quick pulse in a food processor or blender to fluff it back up.
3.　　Using the proportions above, try watermelon and lime juice, cantaloupe and lime juice, or honeydew and orange juice for other refreshing flavor variations.

Spiced Baked Pears with Mascarpone
PREP TIME: 10 MINUTES / COOK TIME: 20 MINUTES/ SERVES 2
Ingredients
2 ripe pears, peeled
1 tablespoon plus 2 teaspoons honey, divided
1 teaspoon vanilla, divided
¼ teaspoon ginger
¼ teaspoon ground coriander
¼ cup minced walnuts
¼ cup mascarpone cheese
Pinch salt
Directions
1.　　**Preparing the Ingredients**
Preheat the oven to 350°F and set the rack to the middle position. Grease a small baking dish.
Cut the pears in half lengthwise. Using a spoon, scoop out the core from each piece. Place the pears with the cut side up in the baking dish.
Combine 1 tablespoon of honey, ½ teaspoon of vanilla, ginger, and coriander in a small bowl. Pour this mixture evenly over the pear halves.
Sprinkle walnuts over the pear halves.
2.　　**Bake**. For 20 minutes, or until the pears are golden and you're able to pierce them easily with a knife.
While the pears are baking, mix the mascarpone cheese with the remaining 2 teaspoons honey, ½ teaspoon of vanilla, and a pinch of salt. Stir well to combine.
Divide the mascarpone among the warm pear halves and serve.
If you don't have ripe pears on hand, try substituting apples. They may need a few more minutes of baking time.

Vanilla Greek Yogurt Affogato
PREP TIME: 10 MINUTES / COOK TIME: NONE/ SERVES 4
Ingredients
24 ounces vanilla Greek yogurt
2 teaspoons sugar

4 shots hot espresso or ¾ cup (6 ounces) strong brewed coffee
4 tablespoons chopped unsalted pistachios
4 tablespoons dark chocolate chips or shavings
Directions
Preparing the Ingredients. Spoon the yogurt into four bowls or tall glasses. Mix ½ teaspoon of sugar into each of the espresso shots (or all the sugar into the coffee). Pour one shot of hot espresso or 1.5 ounces of coffee over each bowl of yogurt. Top each bowl with 1 tablespoon of pistachios and 1 tablespoon of chocolate chips and serve.

Roasted Plums with Nut Crumble
PREP TIME: 5 MINUTES / COOK TIME: 25 MINUTES/ SERVES 4
Ingredients
¼ cup honey
¼ cup freshly squeezed orange juice
4 large plums, halved and pitted
¼ cup whole-wheat pastry flour
1 tablespoon pure maple sugar
1 tablespoon nuts, coarsely chopped (your choice; I like almonds, pecans, and walnuts)
1½ teaspoons canola oil
½ cup plain Greek yogurt
Directions
Preparing the Ingredients
1.　　Preheat the oven to 400°F. Combine the honey and orange juice in a square baking dish. Place the plums, cut-side down, in the dish. Roast about 15 minutes, and then turn the plums over and roast an additional 10 minutes, or until tender and juicy.
2.　　In a medium bowl, combine the flour, maple sugar, nuts, and canola oil and mix well. Spread on a small baking sheet and bake alongside the plums, tossing once, until golden brown, about 5 minutes. Set aside until the plums have finished cooking. Serve the plums drizzled with pan juices and topped with the nut crumble and a dollop of yogurt.

Baked Apples with Walnuts and Spices
PREP TIME: 10 MINUTES / COOK TIME: 45 MINUTES/ SERVES 4
Ingredients
4 apples
¼ cup chopped walnuts
2 tablespoons honey
1 teaspoon ground cinnamon
¼ teaspoon ground nutmeg
¼ teaspoon ground ginger
Pinch sea salt
Directions
Preparing the Ingredients. Preheat the oven to 375°F. Cut the tops off the apples and use a metal spoon or paring knife to remove the cores, leaving the bottoms of the apples intact. Place the apples cut-side up in a 9-by-9-inch baking pan.
In a small bowl, stir together the walnuts, honey, cinnamon, nutmeg, ginger, and sea salt. Spoon the

mixture into the centers of the apples. Bake the apples for about 45 minutes until browned, soft, and fragrant. Serve warm.

Orange Olive Oil Mug Cakes

PREP TIME: 10 MINUTES / COOK TIME: 2 MINUTES/ SERVES 2

Ingredients

6 tablespoons flour
2 tablespoons sugar
½ teaspoon baking powder
Pinch salt
1 teaspoon orange zest
1 egg
2 tablespoons olive oil
2 tablespoons freshly squeezed orange juice
2 tablespoons milk
½ teaspoon orange extract
½ teaspoon vanilla extract

Directions

Preparing the Ingredients. In a small bowl, combine the flour, sugar, baking powder, salt, and orange zest.

In a separate bowl, whisk together the egg, olive oil, orange juice, milk, orange extract, and vanilla extract. Pour the dry ingredients into the wet ingredients and stir to combine. The batter will be thick. Divide the mixture into two small mugs that hold at least 6 ounces each, or one 12-ounce mug. Microwave each mug separately. The small ones should take about 60 seconds, and one large mug should take about 90 seconds, but microwaves can vary. The cake will be done when it pulls away from the sides of the mug.

Grilled Stone Fruit with Whipped Ricotta

PREP TIME: 10 MINUTES / COOK TIME: 10 MINUTES/ SERVES 4

Ingredients

Nonstick cooking spray
4 peaches or nectarines (or 8 apricots or plums), halved and pitted
2 teaspoons extra-virgin olive oil
¾ cup whole-milk ricotta cheese
1 tablespoon honey
¼ teaspoon freshly grated nutmeg
4 sprigs mint, for garnish (optional)

Directions

1.   Preparing the Ingredients

Spray the cold grill or a grill pan with nonstick cooking spray. Heat the grill or grill pan to medium heat.

Place a large, empty bowl in the refrigerator to chill.

2.   Cook.

Brush the fruit all over with the oil. Place the fruit cut-side down on the grill or pan and cook for 3 to 5 minutes, or until grill marks appear. (If you're using a grill pan, cook in two batches.) Using tongs, turn the fruit over. Cover the grill (or the grill pan with aluminum foil) and cook for 4 to 6 minutes, until the

fruit is easily pierced with a sharp knife. Set aside to cool.

Remove the bowl from the refrigerator and add the ricotta. Using an electric beater, beat the ricotta on high for 2 minutes. Add the honey and nutmeg and beat for 1 more minute. Divide the warm (or room temperature) fruit among 4 serving bowls, top with the ricotta mixture, and a sprig of mint (if using) and serve.

Figs with Mascarpone and Honey

PREP TIME: 5 MINUTES / COOK TIME: 5 MINUTES/ SERVES 4

Ingredients

⅓ cup walnuts, chopped
8 fresh figs, halved
¼ cup mascarpone cheese
1 tablespoon honey
¼ teaspoon flaked sea salt

Directions

Preparing the Ingredients

1.   In a skillet over medium heat, toast the walnuts, stirring often, 3 to 5 minutes.

2.   Arrange the figs cut-side up on a plate or platter. Using your finger, make a small depression in the cut side of each fig and fill with mascarpone cheese. Sprinkle with a bit of the walnuts, drizzle with the honey, and add a tiny pinch of sea salt.

Red Wine Poached Pears

PREP TIME: 10 MINUTES / COOK TIME: 45 MINUTES (PLUS 3 HOURS TO CHILL)/ MAKES ½ CUP / SERVES 4

Ingredients

2 cups dry red wine
¼ cup honey
Zest of ½ orange
2 cinnamon sticks
1 (1-inch) piece fresh ginger
4 pears, bottom inch sliced off so the pear is flat

Directions

Preparing the Ingredients

1.   In a large pot over medium-high heat, stir together the wine, honey, orange zest, cinnamon, and ginger. Bring to a boil, stirring occasionally. Reduce the heat to medium-low and simmer for 5 minutes to let the flavors blend.

Add the pears to the pot. Cover and simmer for 20 minutes until the pears are tender, turning every 3 to 4 minutes to ensure even color and contact with the liquid. Refrigerate the pears in the liquid for 3 hours to allow for more flavor absorption.

2.   Bring the pears and liquid to room temperature. Place the pears on individual dishes and return the poaching liquid to the stove top over medium-high heat. Simmer for 15 minutes until the liquid is syrupy. Serve the pears with the liquid drizzled over the top.

You can also poach the pears in a sweet wine. Use 2 cups sweet dessert wine, such as ice wine or Sauternes. Use the same spices; just omit the honey.

Dark Chocolate Bark With Fruit And Nuts

PREP TIME: 15 MINUTES, PLUS 1 HOUR TO COOL / COOK TIME: 25 MINUTES / SERVES 2

Ingredients

2 tablespoons chopped nuts (almonds, pecans, walnuts, hazelnuts, pistachios, or any combination of those)

3 ounces good-quality dark chocolate chips (about ⅔ cup)

¼ cup chopped dried fruit (apricots, blueberries, figs, prunes, or any combination of those)

Directions

Preparing the Ingredients

1.   Line a sheet pan with parchment paper. Place the nuts in a skillet over medium-high heat and toast them for 60 seconds, or just until they're fragrant.

2.   Place the chocolate in a microwave-safe glass bowl or measuring cup and microwave on high for 1 minute. Stir the chocolate and allow any unmelted chips to warm and melt. If necessary, heat for another 20 to 30 seconds, but keep a close eye on it to make sure it doesn't burn.

Pour the chocolate onto the sheet pan. Sprinkle the dried fruit and nuts over the chocolate evenly and gently pat in so they stick.

3.   Transfer the sheet pan to the refrigerator for at least 1 hour to let the chocolate harden. When solid, break into pieces. Store any leftover chocolate in the refrigerator or freezer.

Another way to prepare these is to divide the melted chocolate into mini baking cups. Put the cups into a mini muffin pan, fill each with chocolate, and sprinkle the nuts and fruit on top. Use a toothpick to gently push the fruit and nuts into the chocolate.

Pomegranate-Quinoa Dark Chocolate Bark

PREP TIME: 10 MINUTES / COOK TIME: 5 MINUTES/ SERVES 6

Ingredients

Nonstick cooking spray

½ cup uncooked tricolor or regular quinoa

½ teaspoon kosher or sea salt

8 ounces dark chocolate or 1 cup dark chocolate chips

½ cup fresh pomegranate seeds

Directions

Preparing the Ingredients

1.   In a medium saucepan coated with nonstick cooking spray over medium heat, toast the uncooked quinoa for 2 to 3 minutes, stirring frequently. Do not let the quinoa burn. Remove the pan from the stove, and mix in the salt. Set aside 2 tablespoons of the toasted quinoa to use for the topping.

2.   Break the chocolate into large pieces, and put it in a gallon-size zip-top plastic bag. Using a metal ladle or a meat pounder, pound the chocolate until broken into smaller pieces. (If using chocolate chips, you can skip this step.) Dump the chocolate out of the bag into a medium, microwave-safe bowl and heat for 1 minute on high in the microwave. Stir until the chocolate is completely melted. Mix the toasted quinoa (except the topping you set aside) into the melted chocolate.

3.   Line a large, rimmed baking sheet with parchment paper. Pour the chocolate mixture onto the sheet and spread it evenly until the entire pan is covered. Sprinkle the remaining 2 tablespoons of quinoa and the pomegranate seeds on top. Using a spatula or the back of a spoon, press the quinoa and the pomegranate seeds into the chocolate.

4.   Freeze the mixture for 10 to 15 minutes, or until set. Remove the bark from the freezer, and break it into about 2-inch jagged pieces. Store in a sealed container or zip-top plastic bag in the refrigerator until ready to serve.

Greek Yogurt Chocolate "Mousse" With B'erries

PREP TIME: 15 MINUTES, PLUS 15 MINUTES TO CHILL / COOK TIME: 0 MINUTES/ SERVES 4

Ingredients

2 cups plain Greek yogurt

¼ cup heavy cream

¼ cup pure maple syrup

3 tablespoons unsweetened cocoa powder

2 teaspoons vanilla extract

¼ teaspoon kosher salt

1 cup fresh mixed berries

¼ cup chocolate chips

Directions

Preparing the Ingredients

1.   Place the yogurt, cream, maple syrup, cocoa powder, vanilla, and salt in the bowl of a stand mixer or use a large bowl with an electric hand mixer. Mix at medium-high speed until fluffy, about 5 minutes. Spoon evenly among 4 bowls and put in the refrigerator to set for at least 15 minutes.

2.   Serve each bowl with ¼ cup mixed berries and 1 tablespoon chocolate chips.

APPENDIX : RECIPES INDEX

Flatbread with Olive Tapenade 96
Flounder with Tomatoes and Basil 57
Flourless Chocolate Brownies with Raspberry Balsamic Sauce 99
French Lentil Salad with Parsley and Mint 25
French Lentils with Swiss Chard (Instant pot) 89
Fruit Smoothie 10

G

Garlic and Herb Roasted Grape Tomatoes 97
Garlic-Asparagus Israeli Couscous 89
Garlicky Kale And Parsnips With Soft-Cooked Eggs And Pickled Onions (Instant Pot) 8
Garlicky Kale and Parsnips with Soft-Cooked Eggs and Pickled Onions (Instant Pot) 39
Gnocchi with Creamy Butternut Squash and Blue Cheese Sauce 36
Gorgonzola Sweet Potato Burgers 37
Greek Meatballs 80
Greek Salad 18
Greek Turkey Burger 67
Greek Yogurt Breakfast Parfaits With Roasted Grapes 9
Greek Yogurt Chocolate "Mousse" With B'erries 102
Greek Yogurt–Marinated Chicken Breasts 67
Greek-Style Ground Beef Pita Sandwiches 79
Green beans with Potatoes and Basil (Instant Pot) 42
Grilled Eggplant Stacks 48
Grilled Fish on Lemons 54
Grilled Flank Steak With Grilled Vegetables And Salsa Verde 81
Grilled Mahi-Mahi with Artichoke Caponata 58
Grilled Oregano Chicken Kebabs with Zucchini and Olives 66
Grilled Steak, Mushroom, and Onion Kebabs 80
Grilled Stone Fruit with Whipped Ricotta 101
Grilled Stuffed Portobello Mushrooms 40
Grilled Zucchini with Yogurt and Pomegranate 46
Ground Lamb with Lentils and Pomegranate Seeds 82

H

Hake in Saffron Broth (Instant Pot) 59
Halibut en Papillote with Capers, Onions, Olives, and Tomatoes 64
Halibut in Parchment with Zucchini, Shallots, and Herbs 56
Halibut with Carrots, White Beans, and Chermoula (Instant Pot) 62
Harissa Yogurt Chicken Thighs 69
Hearty Italian Turkey Vegetable Soup 17
Herb-Roasted Turkey Breast 69
Honey Almond–Crusted Chicken Tenders 67
Honey Ricotta with Espresso and Chocolate Chips 99
HUMMUS 13

I

Individual Baked Egg Casseroles 10

Italian Baked Beans 83
Italian Salsa Verde 81
Italian White Bean Salad with Bell Peppers 24

J

Julene's Green Juice 9

K

Kibbeh 76

L

Lamb Meatballs 80
Lebanese Rice and Broken Noodles with Cabbage 87
Lemon and Paprika Herb-Marinated Chicken 72
Lemon and Watermelon Granita 99
Lemon Chicken with Artichokes and Crispy Kale 71
Lemon Farro Bowl with Avocado 88
Lemon Herb-Crusted Pork Tenderloin 81
Lemon Kale with Slivered Almonds 43
Lemon Pesto Salmon 59
Lemon-Thyme Roasted Mixed Vegetables 90
Lemony Garlic Hummus 14
Lentil Bolognese 46
Lentil Soup 28
Lentil Sweet Potato Soup 29

M

Mashed Cauliflower 37
Mashed Chickpea, Feta, And Avocado Toast 10
Mediterranean Breakfast Pizza 12
Mediterranean Chimichurri Skirt Steak 79
Mediterranean Cod Stew 62
Mediterranean Fruit, Veggie, and Cheese Board 13
Mediterranean Lentil Sloppy Joes 36
Mediterranean Lentils and Rice 85
Mediterranean Potato Salad 22
Mediterranean Trail Mix 13
Mediterranean Veggie Pizza with Pourable Thin Crust 94
Melon Caprese Salad 19
Meze Plate with Hummus, Spiced Carrots, and Arugula(Instant Pot) 33
Monkfish with Sautéed Leeks, Fennel, and Tomatoes 64
Moroccan Meatballs 77
Moroccan-Inspired Chickpea Tagine 41
Moroccan-Style Chickpea Soup 31
Mushroom Barley Soup 25
Mushroom Ragù with Parmesan Polenta 38
Mushroom-Leek Tortilla de Patatas 34

N

No-Drain Pasta Alla Norma 96
North African Peanut Stew Over Cauliflower Rice 45
No-Stir Polenta with Arugula, Figs, and Blue Cheese (Instant Pot) 85

O

One-Pan Mushroom Pasta with Mascarpone 44
One-Pan Parsley Chicken and Potatoes 69
One-Pan Tuscan Chicken 73

Orange Cardamom Buckwheat Pancakes 8
Orange Olive Oil Mug Cakes 101
Orzo with Spinach and Feta 87
Orzo-Stuffed Tomatoes 47
Overnight Pomegranate Muesli 11

P

Paella Soup 28
Pan-Roasted Salmon with Gremolata 57
Pan-Seared Scallops with Sautéed Spinach 56
Panzanella 23
Parmesan Zucchini Sticks 41
Pasta Puttanesca 90
Pasta with Pesto 91
Pastina Chicken soup with kale 24
Penne and Fresh Tomato Sauce with Fennel and Orange 91
Penne and Fresh Tomato Sauce with Spinach and Feta 92
Pistachio Mint Pesto Pasta 34
Pistachio Parmesan Kale-Arugula Salad 17
Pistachio Quinoa Salad with Pomegranate Citrus Vinaigrette 17
Pistachio-Crusted Whitefish 53
Pizza with Arugula and Balsamic Glaze 94
Pizza with Red Bell Peppers, Basil, Arugula, and Caramelized Onion 95
Poached Salmon (Instant Pot) 53
Polenta With Sautéed Chard And Fried Eggs 11
Pollock with Roasted Tomatoes 66
Pomegranate-Quinoa Dark Chocolate Bark 102

Q

Quick Toasted Almonds 14
Quickie Honey Nut Granola 10
Quinoa Lentil "Meatballs" With Quick Tomato Sauce 50
Quinoa with Zucchini, Mint, and Pistachios 23

R

Ratatouille 47
Red Gazpacho 27
Red Wine Poached Pears 101
Rice and Spinach 84
Rice Salad with Oranges, Olives, and Almonds 87
Ricotta, Basil, and Pistachio–Stuffed Zucchini 42
Roasted Asparagus Caprese Pasta 97
Roasted Branzino with Lemon and Herbs 64
Roasted Broccoli with Tahini Yogurt Sauce 15
Roasted Broccolini with Garlic and Romano 93
Roasted Brussels Sprouts with Delicata Squash and Balsamic Glaze 95
Roasted Carrot Soup with Parmesan Croutons 27
Roasted Cauliflower and Arugula Salad with Pomegranate and Pine Nuts 26
Roasted Cauliflower With Lemon Tahini Sauce 97
Roasted Eggplant and Chickpeas with Tomato Sauce 49
Roasted Eggplant Soup 29

Roasted Fennel with Tomatoes 44
Roasted Feta with Kale and Lemon Yogurt 48
Roasted Golden Beet, Avocado, and Watercress Salad 21
Roasted Plums with Nut Crumble 100
Roasted Portobello Mushrooms with Kale and Red Onion 40
Roasted Ratatouille Pasta 37
Roasted Red Pepper Soup with Smoked Paprika and Cilantro Yogurt 25
Roasted Tomato Pita Pizzas 90
Romesco Dip 15
Rustic Garlic Toasts with Stewed Tomatoes, Shaved Fennel, and Burrata (Instnt Pot) 35

S

Salmon Burgers 58
Salmon Cakes with Bell Pepper and Lemon Yogurt 54
Salmon Cakes with Tzatziki Sauce 61
Salmon with Garlicky Broccoli Rabe and White Beans (Instant Pot) 55
Salmon with Lemon-Garlic Mashed Cauliflower (Instant Pot) 54
Salmon with Wild Rice and Orange Salad (Instant Pot) 56
Sardine Bruschetta with Fennel and Lemon Crema 61
Sautéed Cabbage with Parsley and Lemon 43
Sautéed Chicken Cutlets with Romesco Sauce 65
Sautéed Kale with Tomato and Garlic 14
Seared Halloumi with Pesto and Tomato 15
Seared Scallops with White Bean Purée 58
Sheet Pan Lemon Chicken and Roasted Artichokes 74
Sheet Pan Roasted Chickpeas and Vegetables with Harissa Yogurt 49
Shrimp Mojo de Ajo 55
Shrimp Scampi 53
Shrimp with Arugula Pesto and Zucchini Noodles 60
Sicilian Fish Stew(Instant Pot) 23
Simple Summer Gazpacho 24
Skillet Creamy Tarragon Chicken and Mushrooms 73
Skillet Greek Turkey and Rice 71
Smoked Salmon Egg Scramble With Dill And Chives 12
Socca Pan Pizza with Herbed Ricotta, Fresh Tomato, and Balsamic Glaze 32
Spaghetti Squash Marinara 51
Spanish Style Turkey Meatball Soup (Instant Pot) 19
Spiced Almonds 15
Spiced Baked Pears with Mascarpone 100
Spiced Couscous 84
Spiced Rice Pilaf with Sweet Potatoes and Pomegranate (Instant Pot) 83
Spiced Winter Squash with Halloumi and Shaved Brussels Sprouts 44

Spicy Lamb Burgers with Harissa Mayo 76
Spicy Sausage Lentil Soup 19
Spicy Wilted Greens with Garlic 91
Steak With Red Wine–Mushroom Sauce 79
Steamed Mussels in White Wine Sauce 63
Strawberry Basil Honey Ricotta Toast 9
Stuffed Cucumber Cups 16
Stuffed Red Bell Peppers 48
Stuffed Tomatoes with Tabbouleh 42
Sumac Chicken with Cauliflower and Carrots 70
Summer Panzanella Salad 23
Summer Squash Ribbons with Lemon and Ricotta 13
Sun-Dried Tomato and Artichoke Pizza 93
Sunny-Side Up Baked Eggs With Swiss Chard, Feta, And Basil 8
Sweet Potato Mash 85
Swordfish Kebabs 61
Swordfish with Peppers and Potatoes (Instant Pot) 63

T

Tabbouleh 86
Tahini Chicken Rice Bowls 72
Three-Bean Vegetable Chili 51
Toasted Orzo with Shrimp and Feta 93
Tourli Greek Baked Vegetables 46
Triple-Green Pasta 95
Turkey Burgers with Mango Salsa 68
Turmeric Red Lentil Soup 30

Tuscan Bean Soup with Kale 30
Tuscan Tuna and Zucchini Burgers 59

V

Vanilla Greek Yogurt Affogato 100
Vegetable Fagioli 20

W

Walnut Pesto Zoodles 33
Watermelon Feta Salad 24
Weeknight Sheet Pan Fish Dinner 56
White Bean Harissa Dip 13
White Bean Soup with Kale 26
White Beans With Rosemary, Sage, And Garlic 98
White Clam Pizza Pie 92
Wild Mushroom Farrotto (Instant Pot) 86
Wild Rice Salad with Chickpeas and Pickled Radish 22
Wine-Braised Short Ribs with Potatoes (Instant Pot) 78

Y

Yogurt With Blueberries, Honey, And Mint 12

Z

Za'atar Chicken Tenders 73
Za'atar Rubbed Chicken with Celery Root and Spinach (Instant Pot) 65
Zucchini and Meatball Soup 30
Zucchini Noodles with Peas and Mint 52
Zucchini With Bow Ties 97
Zucchini-Eggplant Gratin 39

Printed in the USA
CPSIA information can be obtained
at www.ICGtesting.com
LVHW062048090923
757632LV00006B/431